www.ingramcontent.com/pod-product-compliance
Lightning Source LLC
Chambersburg PA
CBHW071148050326
40689CB00011B/2028

I0003213

Tobias Heimann

Statistical Shape Models for 3D Medical Image
Segmentation

Tobias Heimann

# Statistical Shape Models for 3D
# Medical Image Segmentation

VDM Verlag Dr. Müller

## Impressum/Imprint (nur für Deutschland/ only for Germany)

Bibliografische Information der Deutschen Nationalbibliothek: Die Deutsche Nationalbibliothek verzeichnet diese Publikation in der Deutschen Nationalbibliografie; detaillierte bibliografische Daten sind im Internet über http://dnb.d-nb.de abrufbar.

Alle in diesem Buch genannten Marken und Produktnamen unterliegen warenzeichen-, marken- oder patentrechtlichem Schutz bzw. sind Warenzeichen oder eingetragene Warenzeichen der jeweiligen Inhaber. Die Wiedergabe von Marken, Produktnamen, Gebrauchsnamen, Handelsnamen, Warenbezeichnungen u.s.w. in diesem Werk berechtigt auch ohne besondere Kennzeichnung nicht zu der Annahme, dass solche Namen im Sinne der Warenzeichen- und Markenschutzgesetzgebung als frei zu betrachten wären und daher von jedermann benutzt werden dürften.

Coverbild: www.purestockx.com

Verlag: VDM Verlag Dr. Müller Aktiengesellschaft & Co. KG
Dudweiler Landstr. 125 a, 66123 Saarbrücken, Deutschland
Telefon +49 681 9100-698, Telefax +49 681 9100-988, Email: info@vdm-verlag.de
Zugl.: Heidelberg, Uni, Diss., 2008

Herstellung in Deutschland:
Schaltungsdienst Lange o.H.G., Zehrensdorfer Str. 11, D-12277 Berlin
Books on Demand GmbH, Gutenbergring 53, D-22848 Norderstedt
Reha GmbH, Dudweiler Landstr. 99, D- 66123 Saarbrücken
ISBN: 978-3-639-05056-1

## Imprint (only for USA, GB)

Bibliographic information published by the Deutsche Nationalbibliothek: The Deutsche Nationalbibliothek lists this publication in the Deutsche Nationalbibliografie; detailed bibliographic data are available in the Internet at http://dnb.d-nb.de.

Any brand names and product names mentioned in this book are subject to trademark, brand or patent protection and are trademarks or registered trademarks of their respective holders. The use of brand names, product names, common names, trade names, product descriptions etc. even without
a particular marking in this works is in no way to be construed to mean that such names may be regarded as unrestricted in respect of trademark and brand protection legislation and could thus be used by anyone.

Cover image: www.purestockx.com

Publisher:
VDM Verlag Dr. Müller Aktiengesellschaft & Co. KG
Dudweiler Landstr. 125 a, 66123 Saarbrücken, Germany
Phone +49 681 9100-698, Fax +49 681 9100-988, Email: info@vdm-verlag.de

Copyright © 2008 VDM Verlag Dr. Müller Aktiengesellschaft & Co. KG and licensors
All rights reserved. Saarbrücken 2008

Produced in USA and UK by:
Lightning Source Inc., 1246 Heil Quaker Blvd., La Vergne, TN 37086, USA
Lightning Source UK Ltd., Chapter House, Pitfield, Kiln Farm, Milton Keynes, MK11 3LW, GB
BookSurge, 7290 B. Investment Drive, North Charleston, SC 29418, USA
ISBN: 978-3-639-05056-1

# Abstract

The increasing importance of three-dimensional imaging in medicine leads to a growing demand for volumetric image analysis and automatic segmentation. Due to their robust performance, statistical shape models trained on a collection of example data are especially suited for that purpose. In this thesis, a three-step procedure for generating these models and employing them for 3D segmentation was designed and implemented.

The first step is the identification of corresponding landmarks on the example data, required for training the geometric models. This is solved by a local optimization approach which first employs a gradient descent method for 3D correspondence detection. A continuous reconfiguration of landmarks ensures an exact representation of the shape during optimization. The second step consists of modeling the appearance, i.e. gray-value environment, of the object of interest. In order to compare different models with each other and to find optimal parameter values, a performance index for the objective evaluation of appearance models is developed. The final step integrates shape and appearance model into a robust search algorithm to analyze new images. For the first time, a method for optimal surface detection is combined with an iteratively deformable model. In contrast to standard shape models, additional free deformation is allowed, which permits a more accurate adaption to new data.

The presented methods were evaluated on three medical applications: segmentation of the liver in CT data, of the lung in MR data, and of the prostate in ultrasound images. For all three applications, statistical models could be created successfully. The average surface errors of the obtained segmentations are 1.5 mm for the liver, 2.3 mm for the lung, and 1.1 mm for the prostate. Final result of this thesis is a system for fully automated segmentation of 3D images, which given adequate training data is applicable to a wide range of clinical problems and can replace tedious manual segmentation completely in many cases.

# Publications

Some ideas and figures from this thesis have appeared previously in the following publications:

## Peer-reviewed international conferences and journals

- T. Heimann, I. Wolf, and H.-P. Meinzer. Automatic Generation of 3D Statistical Shape Models with Optimal Landmark Distributions. *Methods Inf Med*, 46(3):275–281, 2007.

- T. Heimann, S. Münzing, H.-P. Meinzer, and I. Wolf. A Shape-Guided Deformable Model with Evolutionary Algorithm Initialization for 3D Soft Tissue Segmentation. *Inf Process Med Imaging*, 20:1–12, 2007.

- T. Heimann, I. Wolf, and H.-P. Meinzer. Active Shape Models for a Fully Automated 3D Segmentation of the Liver – an Evaluation on Clinical Data. *Med Image Comput Comput Assist Interv Int Conf Med Image Comput Comput Assist Interv*, 9(Pt 2):41-8, 2006.

- T. Heimann, I. Wolf, and H.-P. Meinzer. Optimal Landmark Distributions for Statistical Shape Model Construction. In *SPIE Medical Imaging 2006: Image Processing*, pages 518–528, 2006.

- T. Heimann, I. Wolf, T. G. Williams, and H.-P. Meinzer. 3D Active Shape Models Using Gradient Descent Optimization of Description Length. *Inf Process Med Imaging*, 19:566–577, 2005.

## Peer-reviewed national conferences

- T. Heimann, S. Münzing, I. Wolf, and H.-P. Meinzer. Freiheit für Formmodelle! In *Bildverarbeitung für die Medizin 2007*, pp. 136–140, Springer, 2007.

- S. Münzing, T. Heimann, I. Wolf, and H.-P. Meinzer. Evaluierung von Erscheinungsmodellen für die Segmentierung mit statistischen Formmodellen. In *Bildverarbeitung für die Medizin 2007*, pp. 277–281, Springer, 2007.

- M. Schönig, T. Heimann, and H.-P. Meinzer. Parametrisierung geschlossener Oberflächen für die Erzeugung von 3D-Formmodellen. In *Bildverarbeitung für die Medizin 2007*, pp. 394–398, Springer, 2007.

- T. Heimann, I. Wolf, and H.-P. Meinzer. Automatische Erstellung von gleichmäßig verteilten Landmarken für statistische Formmodelle. In *Bildverarbeitung für die Medizin 2007*, pp. 136–140, Springer, 2007.

*Meanwhile we have actually succeeded
in making our discipline a science,
and in a remarkably simple way:
merely by deciding to call it "computer science".*

— Donald E. Knuth (1974)

# Acknowledgments

This thesis was prepared and written at the Division of Medical and Biological Informatics at the German Cancer Research Center by the Naturwissenschaftlich-Mathematischen Gesamtfakultät of the University of Heidelberg. During that time, the German Research Foundation DFG paid a major part of my salary, which is hereby gratefully acknowledged.

I would like to thank my colleagues and friends at the department for the great times we had, be it in the office, at conferences or during other activities: our bridge festivals, christmas parties, and conclave meetings are unforgettable memories – at this point, three cheers for Lena's car (sorry, I forgot its name again) and all its passengers. To Daniel, Ingmar, Marco and Matthias, I thoroughly enjoyed our five o'clock Q3 sessions, although it was waaaay too easy sometimes ;–)

Regarding more work-related matters, I'd especially like to thank Ivo for always having an open ear for tricky math problems and more, and Max for the best paper and abstract reviewing in-house. Thanks to Rhodri Davies for answering my MDL-related questions in many helpful e-mails. This thesis was proofread in remarkably short time by Ivo and Tobi, thanks for all your comments and suggestions. Grammar and language were checked by Amanda who tried to get rid of all my "colloquialisms" (apart from this section which I did not show her): thank you.

I would like to thank my boss and head of department Pitt Meinzer for fostering the great atmosphere in our group and giving me so much freedom for this project. Thanks also to Bernd Jähne for accepting the supervision at the University of Heidelberg.

Last but not least, I would like to thank my parents for supporting me over all these years (and it is a looong time by now): Thank you!

# Contents

*Contents*

*Contents*

# List of Figures

# List of Tables

# 1 Introduction

*The best way to become acquainted with a subject
is to write a book about it.*

*— Benjamin Disraeli*

## 1.1 Motivation

Medical image computing has become a key technology in modern medicine [97]. With the establishment of picture archiving and communication
systems (PACS), images from the radiology department are accessible in the
entire clinic, paving the way for formerly exotic applications like computer-
aided diagnosis (CAD), image-guided surgery (IGS) and surgical planning
systems into clinical routine. Technological advances continue to reduce
costs and improve quality of patient care, especially in the domain of digital imaging. Increasingly, images are acquired as three-dimensional volumes, using modalities like 3D-ultrasound (US), magnetic resonance imaging (MRI), computed tomography (CT), or positron emission tomography
(PET). The new technology provides a view into the human body which is
detailed as never before.

However, hundreds of slices, as produced by the latest generation of MRI
and CT scanners, are tedious to analyze on a one-by-one basis. Consequently, the need for three-dimensional visualization and analysis tools is
growing at a fast pace, and with it the need for reliable and accurate segmentation techniques. Segmentation is the fundamental basis of virtually
all computer-based imaging applications in medicine, as it is required for
CAD, IGS, surgical planning, radiotherapy planning and much more.

Spanning the last two decades, model-based segmentation approaches
have been established as one of the most successful methods for image
analysis. By matching a model which contains information about the expected shape and appearance of the structure of interest to new images,

1

segmentation is conducted in a top-down fashion. Due to the inherent a-priori information, this approach is more stable against local image artifacts and perturbations than conventional low-level algorithms. While a single template shape is an adequate model for industrial applications where mass-produced, rigid objects need to be detected, this method is prone to fail in case of biological objects due to their considerable natural variability. Information about common variations must therefore be included in the model. An approach to gather this information is to examine a number of training shapes by statistical means, leading to the technique of statistical shape models (SSMs).

## 1.2 Objectives

Main objective of this work is to develop an SSM-based system for segmentation of various medical structures. The new method should feature the following properties:

- Easily trainable / extendable: for building the statistical model, no human interaction should be required. Moreover, the training process should be reasonably efficient, i.e. it should run on a standard desktop PC in a matter of hours or a couple of days, not longer. This ensures that it is possible to extend the model with new data on a regular basis.

- Robust, accurate and fast performance: although the new method is not expected to reach human-like performance on all images, it should be reasonably robust and deliver segmentations with an accuracy that is usable for real medical tasks. In addition, it should perform fast enough to be included in the clinical workflow – depending on the task, the critical time-limit might range from a couple of minutes to half an hour.

- Generic applicability: the developed method should not be restricted to one or two tasks, but have a wide area of different applications. It should be transferable to new problems with minimum changes, preferably by simply providing new training data.

## 1.3 Structure of this thesis

This thesis is organized as follows: Chapter 2 describes the current state of the art for SSMs in 3D medical imaging. The basic components of statistical models of shape and appearance are presented and various choices to be made are compared. As such, this chapter forms the basis for all the novel work presented in the following chapters.

Chapter 3 describes a new method to construct 3D shape models. In particular, it presents a solution to optimizing point correspondences between different shapes which is more efficient than previous approaches. It also depicts a method to obtain a better geometric representation of the modeled object of interest.

Chapter 4 presents a number of statistical appearance models that locally describe the boundary of modeled objects. It includes various methods using profile models and a new approach based on local histograms. In addition, a novel method to evaluate the performance of different appearance models is presented.

Chapter 5 employs the techniques presented in the previous two chapters to analyze 3D image data. It features a deformable surface model with novel terms for internal and external energies to adapt to new data as accurate as possible. It also presents a global search mechansim based on evolutionary algorithms to initialize the SSM in new images.

Chapter 6 describes the experiments conducted for three different applications of medical imaging. All previously presented methods are evaluated step by step.

Chapter 7 discusses the obtained results in detail, and Chapter 8 concludes the thesis with a summary of contributions and an outlook for future work.

# 2 State of the Art

*All information looks like noise until you break the code.*

— Neal Stephenson, "Snow Crash" (1992)

This chapter reviews methods and procedures for generating, training and employing statistical models of shape and appearance for 3D medical image analysis. Specifically, it discusses work on discrete, parametric models which can be trained from a set of example data. Probably the best-known methods in that area are the Active Shape Models [43] and Active Appearance Models [32] by Cootes et al. In addition, related concepts and alternative approaches are discussed, all within the context of statistical shape models. Due to the constantly increasing importance of 3D imaging and the urgent need for segmentation in that particular area, this survey concentrates on methods for volumetric images. However, many modeling methods have only been applied to 2D so far. To the extent that such methods can be generalized or extended to the 3D case, they have been included in the present review. Furthermore, some methods have been included which have shown to be very successful in 2D, but which are technically not feasible in 3D – simply to emphasize the difference.

In order to present a systematic overview of the topic, this chapter is divided into several parts, each highlighting a specific aspect of statistical shape models. After briefly delineating related work in Sec. 2.1, different possibilities of how to represent shapes for statistical analysis are presented in Sec. 2.2. Subsequently, Sec. 2.3 explains how to extract the principal modes of variation from a set of training shapes. A general requirement for this step is that the correspondences between all shapes of the training set are known, a topic which will be discussed in Sec. 2.4. After that, Sec. 2.5, presents techniques to model the appearance of the examined object. The different algorithms that employ shape and appearance models for image analysis and segmentation will be discussed in Sec. 2.6. To conlcude, an overview of the areas of application in medical imaging which have been tackled with three-dimensional SSMs is presented in Sec. 2.7.

## 2.1 Related work

Before reviewing statistical shape models, this section defines what is regarded as related work that will not be discussed further.

### 2.1.1 Freely deformable models

Kass et al. started the use of deformable models for image analysis in their seminal snakes paper [125]. Their main idea is that model evolution is driven by two energies: an external energy that adapts the model to the image data and an internal energy that stabilizes its shape based on general smoothness constraints. Shortly afterwards, Terzopoulos et al. [238] generalized the concept (which initially had only been applied to 2D examples) to 3D shapes. In [65], Delingette introduced the deformable simplex mesh, which features a stable internal energy that can easily be customized to deform toward a specific template shape. Using a different approach, McInerney and Terzopoulos [165] presented a method of how to implement topology changes for deformable surfaces. After almost two decades of deformable models, several review articles on the topic have been published, notably by McInerney and Terzopoulos [164], Jain et al. [121] and Montagnat et al. [171]. These methods were disregarded in this review because the underlying deformation algorithms do not incorporate learned constraints of shape variability. Although freely-deformable models can be customized to represent specific shapes (and often are), the stabilizing forces or energies are based on general smoothness properties and are not driven by statistical information.

### 2.1.2 Level-sets

Level-sets were introduced by Osher and Sethian [180] and made popular for computer vision and image analysis by Malladi et al. [161]. They feature an implicit shape representation and can be employed with regional or edge-based features. Leventon et al. [148] extended the original energy formulation by an additional term which deforms the contour towards a previously learned shape model. A frequent criticism is that the signed distance maps which the shape model is based on, do not form a linear space, which can lead to invalid shapes if training samples vary too much. Nevertheless, the approach quickly gained popularity and was extended in several directions, among others by Tsai et al. [246] who employ Leventon's modeling method

with a region-based energy functional. Recently, Pohl et al. [197] presented a method of embedding the signed distance maps into the linear LogOdds space, which could solve the modeling problems. To keep this review at a reasonable length, level-set theory and techniques had to be ignored. The conceptual differences between the implicit representation and the discrete models would have required a special treatment for all following sections. For an overview of statistical approaches to level-set segmentation – including prior shape knowledge – the reader is referred to the recent survey by Cremers et al. [46].

## 2.2 Shape representation

The training data for SSMs in the medical field will most likely consist of segmented volumetric images, i.e. binary voxel data. To be able to process these images for model construction, such data must first be transformed into a different representation. The choice of shape representation is the first fundamental decision when designing statistical shape models. Most of the subsequent steps (described in the following sections) depend on this initial decision, and many methods are technically limited to certain representations. Figure 2.1 shows some common shape representations for a hippocampus example.

### 2.2.1 Landmarks and meshes

Probably the simplest and at the same time the most generic method used to represent shapes is a set of points distributed across the surface (which can be extracted from volume data by e.g. the Marching Cubes algorithm). Coordinates for all k points are concatenated to one vector $\mathbf{x}$ that describes the shape:

$$\mathbf{x} = (x_1, y_1, z_1, \ldots, x_k, y_k, z_k)^\mathsf{T} \tag{2.1}$$

In SSM literature, the involved points are often also referred to as *landmarks*, although they do not need to be located at salient feature points as per the common definition for anatomic landmarks. To point out this contradiction, some authors also call them *semi-landmarks*. Often, additional connectivity information between the points is stored to allow for reconstruction of the surface and calculation of normal vectors, which is important for many search algorithms (see Sec. 2.6). A point set with connectivity information is called a *mesh*. Landmarks have been used extensively

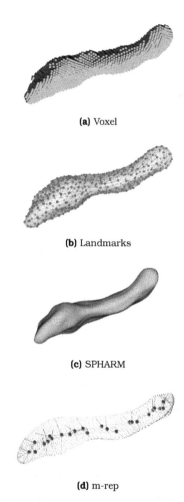

**(a)** Voxel

**(b)** Landmarks

**(c)** SPHARM

**(d)** m-rep

**Figure 2.1:** Different shape representations for the hippocampus, using the original volume data (a), landmarks on a triangulated mesh (b), spherical harmonics (c), and a medial m-rep model (d). All images courtesy by Martin Styner, Neuro Image Analysis Lab, UNC Chapel Hill.

for the statistical study of biological shape by Kendall [129], Bookstein [16] and others. For the use of landmarks as basis of an SSM, Cootes et al. [42] have coined the name *Point Distribution Models* (PDMs), which has become quite popular in literature and is often used synonymously to landmarks. The majority of current shape models are based on PDMs, and they will form a strong focus for the remainder of this article.

### 2.2.2 Medial models

Medial models or skeletons have been used by Blum [14] to describe biological shapes back in the 1970s and are commonly utilized in image analysis. They represent objects by their centerlines and the corresponding radii, often leading to a more compact description than landmarks. Pizer et al. present a medial model with a coarse-to-fine representation for two dimensions in [194]: Basically, it consists of a collection of points on the centerlines and vectors pointing from there toward the boundary. This approach was later extended to 3D in [193] and termed *m-rep*. Recently, Yushkevich et al. [265] presented a continuous version of m-reps. Since their introduction, m-reps have been used successfully for a number of medical image processing tasks, including segmentation, registration and shape discrimination.

### 2.2.3 Other representations

A multitude of other possibilities to represent shape exists, which are only briefly mention here: Staib and Duncan [219] employ Fourier surfaces (an extension of the classical 1D and 2D Fourier transforms) to describe shapes of several different topologies. Closely related is the technique of spherical harmonics (SPHARMs), a set of basis functions which can be used to describe closed surfaces of spherical topology. Among others, this method was employed for deformable models in image analysis by Székely et al. [233] and Kelemen et al. [128]. Matheny and Goldgof [162] present surface harmonics, an extension to SPHARM which can also be used to model non-spherical topologies. Also related to the SPHARM technique is the method employed by Nikou et al. [177] who hierarchically describe surfaces using the vibration modes of a spherical mesh. Another approach for shape description has been proposed by Davatzikos et al. [51], i.e. the use of wavelets. Although their initial paper is only dealing with 2D shape, Nain et al. [174] and Yu et al. [264] recently presented versions using spherical

wavelets for the 3D case. For objects without too many details, non-uniform rational B-Splines (NURBS), as proposed by Tsagaan et al. [245], constitue an efficient shape representation. Here, a small number of control points is sufficient to determine the surface. If the shape information is used for classification purposes only, it is also possible to develop a set of characterizing shape descriptors, as e.g. done by Golland et al. [93]. Last but not least, the level sets approach mentioned in Sec. 2.1.2 is based on an implicit description by signed distance maps. Implicit descriptions can represent arbitrary shapes and inherently support topology changes during deformation.

## 2.3 Shape model construction

Constructing a statistical shape model basically consists of extracting the mean shape and a number of modes of variation from a collection of training samples. Obviously, the methods employed strongly depend on the chosen shape representation. Due to the dominant role of landmark-based point distribution models, this section concentrates on PDMs and only briefly deals with the corresponding procedures for other representations. An essential requirement for building shape models with PDMs is that landmarks on all training samples are located at corresponding positions. The correspondence issue is discussed in detail in Sec. 2.4 – in this section, this requirement is assumed to be fulfilled.

### 2.3.1 Alignment

Shape is defined as a property which does not change under similarity transforms, i.e. it is invariant to translation, rotation and scaling. In general, shape changes induced by these global transforms should not be modeled by an SSM in order to keep the model as specific as possible. For some applications in medical image analysis, however, changes e.g. in size may be treated as part of the biological variation (as done in [175] and [149]). Below, the general case of building a model with similarity transforms removed is assmued. Thus, the first step is to align all training samples in a common coordinate frame.

The most popular method to solve this problem for PDMs is the generalized Procrustes alignment (GPA), as described by Gower [95] and Goodall [94]. The standard Procrustes match (termed after a figure from Greek mythology) minimizes the mean squared distance between two shapes and can be

calculated analytically. To align a group of shapes to their unknown mean, this procedure is run iteratively, resulting in the GPA. In addition to the references provided above, details of the method can also be found in Dryden and Mardia [69]. It should be pointed out that GPA is not resistant to outlier points, and there have been some experiments of replacing the Euclidean distance metric in the scheme with the $L_1$ or $L_\infty$ norm (see Larsen and Eiriksson [143]). Moreover, Ericsson and Karlsson [73] proposed aligning the rotation of all training shapes using Minimum Description Length optimization, similar to the population-based optimization of correspondences (more on this topic in Sec. 2.4.5).

Standard GPA scales all training samples $x_i$ to minimize their Euclidean distance to the mean $\bar{x}$. This procedure leads to non-linearities between the individual shapes which (depending on the amount of variation) will result in inaccuracies in the following decomposition into linear modes of variation. The solution is to project all shapes into the tangent space of the mean by scaling with $1/(x \cdot \bar{x})$. For more information on tangent space, refer to Dryden and Mardia [69]; a short description of the implications for model building is also provided in Cootes and Taylor [41].

## 2.3.2 Dimensionality reduction

After alignment, the next step is to reduce the dimensionality of the training set, i.e. to find a small set of modes that best describes the observed variation. This is usually accomplished using principal component analysis (PCA). Following Eq. 2.1, every aligned training shape is described by 3k point coordinates in the vector $\mathbf{x_i}$. The mean shape can then be formed by simply averaging over all $s$ samples:

$$\bar{\mathbf{x}} = \frac{1}{s} \sum_{i=1}^{s} \mathbf{x_i} \tag{2.2}$$

The corresponding covariance matrix S is given by:

$$S = \frac{1}{s-1} \sum_{i=1}^{s} (\mathbf{x_i} - \bar{\mathbf{x}})(\mathbf{x_i} - \bar{\mathbf{x}})^\mathsf{T} \tag{2.3}$$

An eigendecomposition on S delivers the $(s-1)$ principal modes of variation $\phi_m$ (eigenvectors) and their respective variances $\lambda_m$ (eigenvalues) – Fig. 2.2 visualizes the three largest modes for the example of a liver SSM. Instead of using eigenanalysis on the covariance matrix, it is also possible to calculate $\phi_m$ and $\lambda_m$ by a singular value decomposition (SVD) on the aligned

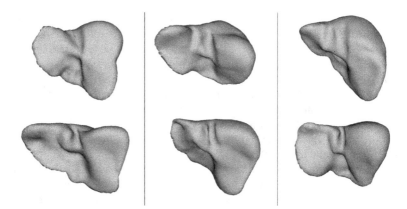

**Figure 2.2:** Principal modes of variation for an SSM of the liver: The left column shows the variation of the largest eigenmode between $\pm 3\sqrt{\lambda_1}$, the medium and right column show the variation of the second and third largest eigenmode, respectively.

landmark matrix $L = ((\mathbf{x_1} - \bar{\mathbf{x}}) \dots (\mathbf{x_s} - \bar{\mathbf{x}}))$. >From a computational point of view, this method is to be preferred due to the higher numerical stability. As both methods set up their principal modes according to least-squares estimation, they are susceptible to outliers – sometimes an entire sample might be outside the expected distribution, sometimes only a small number of landmarks for a given sample. One algorithm that is able to handle both types of outliers is the robust PCA presented by de la Torre and Black [63].

In any case, the resulting modes of variation are ordered by their variances so that $\lambda_1 \geqslant \lambda_2 \geqslant \dots \geqslant \lambda_{s-1}$. In a next step, it is possible to approximate every valid shape by a linear combination of the first c modes:

$$\mathbf{x} = \bar{\mathbf{x}} + \sum_{m=1}^{c} b_m \phi_m \tag{2.4}$$

In many cases, c is chosen so that the accumulated variance $\sum_{m=1}^{c} \lambda_m$ reaches a certain ratio r of the total variance $\sum_{m=1}^{s-1} \lambda_m$. Common values for r are 0.9 to 0.98.

Vector **b** in Eq. 2.4 holds the shape parameters. To constrain the allowed variation to plausible shapes, **b** has to be limited to a certain interval. A common method is to treat all modes as independent distributions and constrain each $b_m$ to lie inside $[-3\lambda_m, 3\lambda_m]$. Alternatively, viewing all modes

as one multi-variate distribution, **b** can also be constrained to lie inside a hyperellipsoid, i.e.

$$\left( \sum_{m=1}^{c} \frac{b_m^2}{\lambda_m} \right) \leqslant M_t \tag{2.5}$$

where $M_t$ is a threshold chosen from the $\chi^2$ distribution. If the shape variation does not follow a Gaussian distribution, the presented constraints for **b** will possibly result in invalid shapes. A more accurate estimate of valid parameter constellations can be obtained by Gaussian mixture models, as proposed by Cootes and Taylor [38]. Recently, Li and Ito [153] presented a method of parameter restriction which is based on multi-dimensional tables that are constructed from the training data.

In general, PCA results in global modes which influence all variables simultaneously, i.e. varying one mode will affect all landmarks of the shape model. For models used for shape analysis or diagnostic purposes, it is usually beneficial to have more isolated effects, which are more intuitive to interpret: Each mode should only affect a limited, preferably locally clustered number of landmarks. This property is called sparsity: a straight-forward method to obtain sparser modes is to employ the Orthomax rotation as proposed by Stegmann et al. [224]. As the name indicates, Orthomax rotates the PCA modes to increase sparsity, while maintaining the orthogonality of components and thus Euclidean space. If the latter property is not essential, sparse PCA by Sjöstrand et al. [215] is an alternative approach which still produces near-orthogonal components. Other decomposition methods do not incorporate any orthogonality criteria at all but directly strive to maximize sparsity. The most popular one is probably the independent component analysis (ICA) [119], which does not assume a Gaussian data distribution and delivers statistically independent projections. Among others, it was applied to shape modeling by Üzümzü et al. [249] and Suinesiaputra et al. [231] for the characterization of myocardial diseases. Another technique to obtain sparse modes of variation is the maximum autocorrelation factor (MAF) analysis as used by Hilger et al. [107]. An extensive comparison between PCA, MAF and minimum noise fraction (MNF – another non-Euclidean decomposition) is presented by Larsen and Hilger [144]. They also prove that MAF is actually equivalent to ICA.

As the non-PCA approaches for dimensionality reduction deliver modes that are not directly specified by variance, there is no natural ordering for these modes. In order to still be able to make a sensible selection of modes

for the SSM, a number of different techniques can be employed [224, 215, 249]. When using non-orthogonal decompositions, it is important to realize that standard methods for shape fitting by least squares projection do no longer work, thus impacting on the model search algorithms (Sec. 2.6).

Apart from exploring different linear decompositions, there has also been work on building non-linear SSMs. Non-linear models allow for natural representation of variations based on bending and rotations, which can only inadequately be approximated by linear models. Sozou et al. suggested non-linear PCA based on polynomial regression [217] and multi-layer perceptrons [218] for this purpose. Later, Twining and Taylor [248] proposed the use of Kernel PCA instead, which they claim to be more general than other methods.

### 2.3.3 Enlarging variations

The power of a statistical model rises and falls with the quantity of available training data. In case of 3D SSMs, this quantity is almost always too low, as in practice there are rarely enough training images available and their required manual segmentation is very cumbersome and time-consuming. This results in models that are over-constrained, i.e. the restrictions imposed on the deformations do not enable them to adapt accurately to new data.

Cootes and Taylor [36] use finite element methods to calculate vibrational modes for each training shape, which are used to generate a number of modified shape instances. All variants are subsequently included in the construction of the SSM, which leads to a model featuring original and synthetic variations. Depending on the amount of original training data, it is possible to adapt the number of generated synthetic shapes. In a subsequent publication [37], the authors present a simpler technique for the same purpose: The synthetic variation is added directly to the covariance matrix $S$, coupling the movement of neighboring points. The same method is used by Wang and Staib [261] to build more flexible models. Lötjönen et al. [159] propose several additional methods of how to synthetically modify training shapes. >From their set, the best results are delivered by a non-rigid movement strategy which deforms shapes randomly by local warping.

A different approach to increase model flexibility is to divide the SSM into several, independently modeled parts. The rationale behind this is that smaller parts exhibit less variation, which can be captured with fewer training samples than the variation for the full shape. For the segmentation of

aortic aneurysms, de Bruijne et al. [61] model cross-sections of the vessel by one SSM, while variations along the axis are captured by a second model. Davatzikos et al. [51] employ the wavelet transform to organize their model into a hierarchy of several parts: The lower bands of the transform correspond to more global shape changes, the higher bands to more local ones. Each band is modeled independently from the other ones. Another modeling scheme based on mesh partitioning is subsequently presented by Zhao et al. [271]: Again, each part of the mesh is modeled separately, but parameters for the individual parts are connected by curves in a combined shape space. The authors claim that limiting these curves to similar patterns as encountered in the training set helps to prevent invalid shapes of the SSM.

## 2.4 Shape correspondence

Modeling the statistics of a class of shapes requires a set of appropriate training shapes with well-defined correspondences. Depending on the chosen representation, the methods of how to best define these correspondences vary. In any case, establishing dense point correspondences between all shapes of the training set is generally the most challenging part of 3D model construction, and at the same time one of the major factors influencing model quality (the other one being the local gray-value appearances). Even for 2D models, manual landmarking is getting increasingly unpopular, not only due to the tedious and time-consuming expert work required, but also due to the lack of reproducibility of the results. In 3D, these arguments weight even heavier, since typically, a much larger amount of landmarks is needed and the correspondences are much harder to pinpoint on 3D shapes – even for experts.

In principle, all algorithms that automatically compute correspondences actually perform a registration between the involved shapes. In this section, all methods have been categorized according to the type of registration process involved, i.e. matching a mesh to another mesh is one category, matching a mesh to an image volume another etc.

### 2.4.1 Mesh-to-mesh registration

The straightforward solution to landmark creation in 3D is to work directly on the training meshes. Figure 2.3 shows the general outline of this

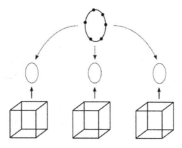

**Figure 2.3:** Basic scheme for mesh-to-mesh registration to determine point correspondences: First, surfaces are extracted from all training images. In a next step, a landmarked template mesh is fitted to all these surfaces, propagating its landmarks to all samples.

scheme. A number of established algorithms exists for surface matching, popular ones being the Iterative Closest Point (ICP) algorithm by Besl and McKay [12] and the Softassign Procrustes by Rangarajan et al. [200]: Both accept two surfaces with potentially different number of vertices as input and deliver the optimal similarity transformation from one surface to the other as a result. Many of the simpler methods of determining correspondences for SSMs directly rely on these algorithms, e.g. by choosing an arbitrary shape as reference and registering it to all others, thus creating all necessary landmarks [104, 257, 123]. One of the shortcomings of this approach is the bias induced by the choice of reference shape – even if the procedure is repeated a second time with the mean shape as reference, as suggested by Vos et al. [257]. A solution to this problem is the method described by Brett and Taylor in [21], based on the ideas published by Hill et al. [111]: A symmetric version of the ICP is used to build a binary tree of well-matching shapes, and landmarks are propagated from the root to the leaves. As pointed out by Frangi et al. [82], this method requires that all possible combinations of matches are scored in advance, but the extra work seems well worth in light of the gained independence from reference shapes. Another improvement to this class of correspondence detection is modification of the similarity metric of the point matching algorithm to include additional features like crest lines (Subsol et al. in [230]), normal vectors (Brett and Taylor in [22]) or local shape and pattern information (Caunce and Taylor in [27]).

The largest draw-back of using a standard point matching algorithm like ICP for landmark creation is the restriction to similarity transformations. While this may be sufficient to match relatively similar training shapes such as bones, it is not adequate for a population of shapes featuring larger variations: In such cases, determination of corresponding points by proximity alone can not only lead to obviously wrong correspondences, but also to non-homeomorphic mappings and thus to flipping triangles in the mesh. Among the first to propose non-rigid registration of training meshes for building SSMs were Subsol et al. [230] using B-Splines and Fleute et al. [77] using multi-resolution Octree splines [234]. An alternative to spline-based registration is finding a certain number of matching shape features on all meshes and mapping the other points by methods assuring a homeomorphism: Shelton [209] developed a multi-resolution approach to match a number of surfaces by minimizing a cost function based on similarity, structure and prior information. In [260], Wang et al. match a limited number of landmarks by local surface geometry and determine the other points by geodesic interpolation. Yet another possibility is to use pattern recognition techniques to determine correspondences: Ferrarini et al. [75] determine interesting parts of a surface by way of unsupervised clustering and use a classifier similar to self-organizing-maps to detect the corresponding parts on other shapes. The approach presented by Pitiot et al. [191] uses dynamic programming and pattern matching to find corresponding points according to features learned from a set of sparsely annotated training examples. The work looks very promising, but while the authors claim that it works in arbitrary dimensions, examples are only given for 2D and it is not clear how the method generalizes to surfaces.

If a sparse set of user-generated landmarks is available, these known correspondences can be used to guide a Thin-Plate-Spline deformation as initial registration [157, 118, 184, 185]. However, in order to match the surfaces exactly, an additional step is needed: The simplest solution is to match the spatially closest points [118, 184], but this can lead to non-homeomorphic mappings and again to flipping triangles. For this reason, correspondences should be regularized somehow: Possibilities include mesh relaxation with mass-spring-models as proposed by Lorenz and Krahnstöver [157] or using Markov Random Fields to regularize the deformation field as suggested by Paulsen and Hilger in [185]. In any case, some 10–20 landmarks have to be specified manually on each training shape beforehand – depending on the complexity of shapes and number of samples this might either be relatively easy to accomplish or next to unfeasible.

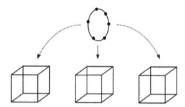

**Figure 2.4:** Basic scheme for mesh-to-volume registration to determine point correspondences: A landmarked deformable surface is adapted to all training images, either to the segmented binary versions or to the original gray-level data. The final positions of landmarks in the images then determine the correspondences.

## 2.4.2 Mesh-to-volume registration

The 3D SSMs in the medical imaging area are almost exclusively based on imaging modalities such as CT, MRI, or 3D-US, i.e. the original data representation of the training shapes is not a mesh but rather a segmented volume. Therefore, a different approach to landmark generation is adapting a deformable surface model to these volumes. The correspondences are then defined by the vertex locations of the deformable template after the surface evolution has converged. Refer to Fig. 2.4 for a schematic illustration of the method. Mostly, the template is fitted to the segmented binary volumes [210, 126, 207, 272], but Fleute et al. [76] and Heitz et al. [106] also use the template to segment the original volume while determining correspondences. This has the advantage that training images do not have to be segmented manually in advance, while it is obviously limited to structures that can be segmented reliably using templates, like e.g. certain bone structures. The deformable surface model is usually extracted from an arbitrary training sample, which can lead to biased results. To minimize this bias, Zhao et al. [272] test beforehand which sample is best-suited as a template and use additional intermediate meshes to segment the data sets for which the standard template did not work adequately. The key to a successful landmark generation using mesh-to-volume registration is the robustness of the deformable template algorithm. Techniques used to ensure the necessary robustness include multi-resolution approaches (Fleute et al. in [76]), gradient vector flow (Shang and Dossel in [207]) and regularizing internal energies (Shen et al. in [210], Kauss et al. in [126] and Zhao et al. in [272]). If the template does not fold itself in the adaptation process, a homeomorphic mapping between the input shapes is guaranteed.

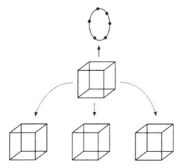

**Figure 2.5:** Basic scheme for volume-to-volume registration to determine point correspondences: A volumetric atlas is matched to all training images, either to the segmented binary versions or to the original gray-level data. The resulting deformation field is used to transform a landmarked template mesh (extracted from the atlas) to all samples, propagating landmarks and defining correspondences.

### 2.4.3 Volume-to-volume registration

Instead of adapting a template mesh to the training data, it is also possible to register a volumetric atlas. Using the resulting deformation field, landmarks placed on the atlas (e.g. by decimating a dense surface mesh) can be propagated to the training data to define the correspondences for the SSM. A visualization of the basic scheme is presented in Fig. 2.5. Frangi et al. describe how to build an atlas of binary volumes using quasi-affine registration with the normalized mutual information (NMI) metric in [82]. Subsequently, a quasi-affine registration followed by a multi-resolution B-Splines deformation is used to warp the atlas to the binary training volumes. In [83], the authors change the underlying NMI to label consistency and Kappa metric to apply the method for multiple objects. In a later publication [178], this version of the algorithm has been tested on 450 input shapes from cardiac MRI with good results – although the volumetric registration does not guarantee a homeomorphic mapping, no triangle flipping was observed.

As with the mesh-to-volume registration, there has also been work on registering a volumetric atlas to the original gray-value images, i.e. without the need for manual segmentations. Rueckert et al. [204] use multi-resolution B-Splines and the NMI metric for that purpose, although they do not propagate landmarks to the training data but perform the statistics on the de-

formation field (the control points of the B-Splines transform) directly. To remove the bias inherent in the atlas construction scheme as per [82], the authors also present a "natural coordinate system" that minimizes deformations from the atlas to the training images. Similar work to establish correspondences is presented by Park et al. [183] using Thin-Plate-Splines and the mutual information metric and Heitz et al. [105] using B-Splines and NMI. The latter two simply use a single representative shape as atlas – obviously with a larger bias than the method by Rueckert et al. [204]. Again, it needs to be emphasized that results of methods working on the original gray volumes strongly depend on the type of objects to be modeled and on the quality of input images. Generally, the more similar the different training samples are and the stronger the objects of interest stand out from the background, the more accurate the resulting statistical models will be.

### 2.4.4 Parameterization-to-parameterization registration

Parameterization is a bijective mapping between a mesh and an appropriate base domain. In 2D, the common base domain for closed contours is the circle, and registering two contours by their parameterization is equivalent to determining correspondences by the relative arc-length. In 3D, parameterization of surfaces is far more complex and usually dependant on the topology of the shape. Most of the methods described below are limited to orientable closed 2D-manifolds of genus zero (i.e. objects without holes and self-intersections), whose common base domain is the sphere. For an introduction to mesh parameterization, refer to Floater and Hormann [78, 79]. Figure 2.6 shows the general outline of the approach for building shape models.

In order to determine correspondences for an SSM, Kelemen et al. [128] propose to generate a spherical harmonics (SPHARM) mapping for each training shape. After aligning all shapes by their first order ellipsoid, the surface points that map to the same position on the sphere are considered to be corresponding. Brett et al. [22] use a similar method for 3D topological disks. In their approach, all shapes are mapped to 2D disks and aligned by optimizing the disk rotation to minimize distances between corresponding points as found by a preceding ICP. While these methods guarantee a diffemorphism between all shapes, the obtained correspondences are mostly arbitrary and the quality of the resulting SSM will depend strongly on the input shapes.

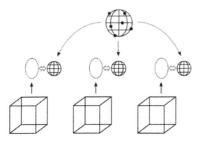

**Figure 2.6:** General outline of the parameterization approach to determine point correspondences: After extracting surfaces from all training images, a one-to-one mapping to a common base domain is created for each surface. By defining landmarks in the base domain, the corresponding points can directly by transferred to all training surfaces using the inverse of the mapping function.

For this reason, other authors have tried to control the parameterizations through a limited set of known or at least assumed correspondences: In order to construct a statistical model of the brain, Thompson et al. [242] manually outline all sulci and transform each resulting parallel cross-section of the surface to a separate parametric mesh. In a similar way, Lamecker et al. [136] let the user specify corresponding patches across different liver shapes, which are again parameterized independently from each other. Praun et al. [198] use harmonic maps to interpolate between a set of corresponding points, either detected by automatic feature comparison or created manually. While these methods explicitly build the parameterizations to conform to the given features, it is also possible to start with standard parameterizations and to subsequently modify them for a better match – a technique also known as re-parameterization. For this purpose, Thompson et al. [243] propose a warping mechanism for spherical maps that matches user-drawn feature lines. Meier and Fisher [167] employ a similarity criterion based on Euclidean point-to-point distances, normal vectors and curvature to guide their warps. Last but not least, Wang et al. [258] calculate curvature features over all training surfaces and optimize a mutual information metric on the corresponding parameterizations. All shapes are automatically divided into the required number of patches, which makes the method independent of the topological genus.

### 2.4.5 Population-based optimization

The first method of determining a population-based (or group-wise) correspondence between shapes was published by Kotcheff and Taylor [135]. Since there was (and still is) no general definition of "ood correspondence" between shapes that could unconditionally be used for pair-wise matching, they focused on the desired properties of the resulting statistical model instead, which they wanted to be as compact as possible, i.e. featuring low eigenvalues concentrated into few modes. To quantify this property, they developed an objective function F based on the determinant of the covariance matrix S (from Eq. 2.3):

$$F = \ln |S + \delta I| - n \ln \delta, \tag{2.6}$$

where I is the identity matrix, n the number of training samples and $\delta$ the amount of additional Gaussian noise. The latter is necessary to prevent problems with zero eigenvalues of S: Since $|S| = \prod \lambda_i$, a single zero leads to an undefined value of F. In their work, Kotcheff and Taylor use a genetic algorithm to modify landmark positions and to minimize F. Although their approach to landmark modification only works in 2D, the core of the approach (i.e. optimization of the objective function) is independent of the number of dimensions. While the method produced good results (in some cases better than manually landmarked models), there were a couple of problems: The genetic optimization scheme did not converge in all cases, the landmark locations had to be chosen from a limited set of points and last but not least, there was no sound theoretical foundation of the objective function.

To remedy the latter issue, Davies et al. proposed a new objective function based on the minimum description length (MDL) of the statistical model [56]. MDL is a principle from information theory which states that the best model should describe the (training) data as efficiently as possible. It runs in line with the principle of Occam's Razor that the simplest solution should be preferred over more complex ones. The full objective function for this approach is a rather complex formula and best described in [52]. Initially, Davies et al. used a piece-wise linear, recursive parameterization scheme to place landmarks and a genetic algorithm to optimize correspondences [56]. Although it was used for 2D only, there was already an outline of how this scheme could be ported to 3D. Later, they switched to a continuous re-parameterization with Cauchy kernels and an optimization using the Nelder-Mead algorithm [53]. The presented results were excellent,

and an extension to the case of 3D objects was finally presented in [55]. The main contribution here was a re-parameterization scheme for closed surfaces of spherical topology (genus-zero), which was implemented using Theta transformations with wrapped Cauchy kernels. Tests on small-sized training sets of brain ventricles and rat kidneys delivered good results and generated further interest in the method.

While the MDL cost function has a sound theoretical foundation, the actual calculation is not trivial and computationally expensive. In [239], Thodberg proposes a simplified version of the cost function:

$$F = \sum_m \mathcal{L}_m \quad \text{with} \quad \mathcal{L}_m = \begin{cases} 1 + \log(\lambda_m/\lambda_{cut}) & \text{for } \lambda_m \geqslant \lambda_{cut} \\ \lambda_m/\lambda_{cut} & \text{for } \lambda_m < \lambda_{cut} \end{cases} \quad (2.7)$$

Although strictly speaking, this version is no MDL and indeed similar to Kotcheff's original formulation (see Eq. 2.6), its performance is comparable to the full MDL and it has gained considerable popularity – last but not least due to the included open source Matlab code for the 2D case. In another paper, Thodberg also suggests to add curvature costs to the objective function [240], but the method is evaluated only on one dataset of 2D face contours.

Whereas the objective function of Eq. 2.7 is simple to compute, the optimization scheme using the Nelder-Mead algorithm is slow and can take hours or days to converge, depending on the number of used landmarks and dimension. While in theory, model-building is only performed once, in practice, tests, optimization and evaluation require a whole number of runs. In [72], Ericsson and Åström derive the gradients of the simplified MDL and present a gradient descent optimization of 2D shapes. As a comparison with the algorithm from [239] reveals, this leads not only to faster convergence but also to better final results.

Whereas re-parameterization on the sphere currently is the most popular method for group-wise correspondence, there are also some alternative approaches: Horkaew et al. [115] parameterize genus-zero shapes to a disc and use piecewise bilinear maps to optimize the MDL criterion. In an evaluation with 38 human left ventricles and a B-Spline shape representation, the method works well, but no comparison with [55] is conducted. In [26], Cates et al. present an approach that optimizes correspondences based on the entropy of shapes (generally equivalent to MDL). They use a non-parametric particle system to place landmarks, which makes the method independent from the topology of the surfaces. Results in 2D surpass the

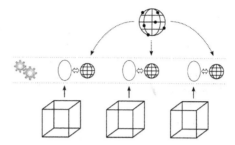

**Figure 2.7:** General outline of an optimization scheme to determine point correspondences: As in the parameterization approach, mappings to a common base
domain are created for all training meshes, and landmarks are defined in the base
domain. In an iterative optimization the mapping functions are modified, resulting in changing correspondences. This process is continued until a cost function
describing the quality of the model has converged to the best value.

simplified MDL optimization from [239], the 3D results look very promising
but have not been compared to other methods yet. Last but not least, there
is work towards a group-wise registration of images by Twining and Cootes
et al. [247, 45]. Until now, the method has only been applied to 2D images,
but it is claimed to be straight-forward to extend to 3D. An outline of the
general scheme to determine point correspondences by optimization (via
parameterizations) is presented in Fig. 2.7.

### 2.4.6 Evaluation of correspondence methods

Given the wide variety of correspondence methods, an objective comparison between them should be capable of differentiating between suitable
and unsuitable approaches. However, this evaluation is hampered by the
fact that the true correspondences of biological shapes are generally not
known. Davies [52] therefore introduced three measures to evaluate the
general quality of an SSM: Generalization ability, specificity and compactness. Generalization ability quantifies the capability of the model to represent new shapes. It can be estimated by performing a series of leave-one-
out tests on the training set, measuring the distance of the omitted training
shape to the closest match of the reduced model. Specificity describes the
validity of the shapes produced by the model. The value is estimated by
generating random parameter values from a normal distribution with zero
mean and the respective standard deviation from the PCA. The distance of

the generated shape to the closest match of the training set is averaged over a large number of runs. Compactness simply measures the accumulative variance of the model. All measures are commonly defined as functions of the number of modes or parameters used by the model and displayed as piecewise linear graphs. Smaller values indicate better models.

Styner et al. [228] employ these three measures to compare models built by manually initialized subdivision surfaces, SPHARM parameterization, and optimization of the determinant of the covariance matrix (Eq. 2.6) and of the MDL. In this comparison, using lateral brain ventricle and femoral head data, the two optimization approaches generate the best results. Another comparison between different correspondence methods is conducted by van Assen in [250]: A heart ventricle model is built using a slice-wise ray-shooting technique and volume-to-volume registration (from Frangi et al. [83]), the latter with two different landmark distributions on the atlas. In addition to the three theoretic measures, the segmentation accuracy of the resulting model on test data is also evaluated. The model built with one of the registration methods reaches the best results for the segmentation task (with only slightly better accuracy than the other two). Remarkably, the synthetic measures for this method result in worse values than for any of the other two.

In another set of experiments, Ericsson and Karlsson [74] also encounter problems with the three measures: In a test with synthetic shapes, models with optimal correspondences score worse results for specificity than those with slightly altered correspondences. The authors therefore propose to use a ground truth correspondence measure, which describes the differences to manual reference landmarks (or the optimal landmarks for synthetic shapes). However, all conducted experiments are performed with 2D shapes and the method seems difficult to transfer to 3D because of excessive manual landmarking.

A first evaluation of different correspondence methods for shape analysis is presented in a recent publication by Styner et al. [229]: Using volumetric registration, SPHARM and MDL optimization, they generate hippocampus models for schizophrenia patients and for a control group. An analysis of the resulting group differences reveals that the utilized correspondence method noticeably influences the results, with the volumetric registration producing the least significant group differences.

## 2.5 Appearance models

The majority of published works uses shape models for image analysis, i.e. after construction the model is fitted to new, previously unseen data. For this purpose, a model of the appearance of the structure of interest is required. Although the first version of shape models simply adapted to the strongest edges in the image [43], the state of the art quickly developed towards specialized, statistical models of appearance. As the shape model, these appearance models have to be trained from sample data. Below, a number of different appearance models based on boundary and region features are presented. In addition, some clustering methods applicable to make the appearance models more robust are highlighted.

### 2.5.1 Boundary-based features

The first statistical appearance models are described by Cootes et al. in [34, 35]: Their basic idea is to sample profiles perpendicular to the surface in all training images and – similar to the shape model construction – extract the mean profile and principal modes of variation for each landmark. During search, the fit of a profile model at a certain position is evaluated by measuring the Mahalanobis distance between the sample profile and the model – in case the complete covariance matrix is not stored, the Mahalanobis distance can be approximated by the largest eigenmodes. Typically, the used profiles contain the plain pixel intensity values, the corresponding derivatives, or the normalized versions thereof. An evaluation of different profile types for face recognition showed that normalized derivative profiles deliver the best results [34]. During another, more extensive evaluation for bone detection in radiographs, the normalized intensity profile generated the most accurate segmentations [9]. While the latter study also reports some experiments with different cost functions (including the correlation coefficient), the Mahalanobis distance generated the best results overall.

It is also possible to combine several different profile types into one large feature vector, as e.g. shown by Brejl et al. [20]: Intensity and gradient profiles are joined with the average inside and outside gray value, and the weighting between different features is handled by the covariance matrix. Another innovative aspect of that study is that intensity profiles are constructed by averaging a number of pixels in the neighborhood, increasing the robustness of the method.

One feature that has been used successfully in face recognition with 2D SSMs is that of Gabor wavelets [49]: This method measures the local image response to a set of Gabor filters, resulting in a feature vector (also called jet) containing amplitude and phase for each individual filter. McKenna et al. [166] were the first to use this Gabor jet in conjunction with a PDM for a video tracking application. The training, however, was limited to the first video frame, where landmarks had to be placed manually. Jiao et al. [122] present a real training method for a set of images, modeling the Gabor jet as a Gaussian mixture model that is created using the EM algorithm [66]. Like McKenna et al., they make use of the fact that the optimal displacement for a landmark can be estimated from the phase information in the corresponding jet. Last but not least, Shen et al. [212] utilize rotation-invariant Gabor filters as smoothing edge detectors for the segmentation of 2D ultrasound images. Since wavelets can also be used in 3D volumes [172], this method seems promising for the analysis of medical data as well. Another type of local descriptor – steerable filters [85] – is utilized by Langs et al. [140]: Like wavelets, this method too can be applied to 3D and might become of interest in medical image analysis.

Relatively early-on in the development of SSMs and appearance models, Haslam et al. [98] presented a Bayesian approach to modeling the boundary appearance, concentrating all landmark profiles from a training image into a single feature vector. Two appearance models are built using the classical method of PCA on the covariance matrix of these feature vectors: The first is a boundary model of the true landmark positions, and the second is a background model created by varying the pose parameters of the training shapes, thereby moving the landmarks to incorrect positions. A downside to this method of modeling the appearance is that due to the concatenation of profiles, it is not possible to independently evaluate the goodness of fit for each landmark, but for the entire shape only. Therefore, the method requires a special form of search algorithms (see also Sec. 2.6) and has not become very popular.

One problem common to all appearance models based on the covariance matrix is that training data (i.e. the profiles) should ideally have a Gaussian distribution. As noted by de Bruijne et al. [60], this is not the case with many medical imaging tasks. As an alternative, a non-linear method to model the object boundary using a kNN-classifier has been proposed: During training, profiles are sampled at the true boundary positions and at a number of additional positions shifted towards the inside and the out-

side of the object. During search, the amount of true profiles among the k nearest neighbors of a sample profile serves as an estimate for the goodness of fit and assumes the role of the Mahalanobis distance. In general, any classifier that calculates a probability value for class membership can be used for that purpose, and not just kNN. Boosting methods, which combine several weak classifiers into a single strong one, are becoming more and more popular, especially the AdaBoost algorithm presented by Freund and Schapire [86]. This algorithm is also used by Li et al. [152] who have trained it on more than 6,000 features calculated by steerable filters. During model search, 200 features per landmark are used at most in order to estimate the probability of points along the normal vector forming part of the boundary. Other approaches employing AdaBoost are presented by Li and Ito [153] who work with a histogram classifier trained on quantized intensity profiles and by Zhang et al. [268] who use Haar wavelets.

Instead of a complete training from sample images, some authors prefer to explicitly specify the boundary appearance: Bailleul et al. [4] calculate four features along each profile, which are assumed to accurately describe the border (of the putamen in MRI datasets): maximum intensity difference between inside and outside voxels, intensity means difference, inner voxels regularity and inner-outer voxels regularity difference. All features are normalized to [0..1] and added to give a final estimate of the boundary fit. In the work of Lamecker et al. [137], all profile intensities on the inside of the modeled shape (a liver in CT datasets) are required to lie within a fixed interval. A preceding diffusion filtering ensures that all intensities are as homogeneous as possible. Similarly, Peters et al. [189] also require certain features (e.g. central gray value, gradient magnitude) to be part of a specific interval. The innovative part of their work is that the interval borders are optimized for each appearance model during a simulated search which estimates the performance of different models.

### 2.5.2 Region-based features

The most popular method using region-based features is the use of Active Appearance Models (see Sec. 2.6.3 for details). Here, the entire inner region of the shape model is employed to build a feature vector $\mathbf{g}$, in the simplest case by storing the plain intensity values of all pixels of the region, i.e. the image texture. To build $\mathbf{g}$ for different shapes, the respective region has to be transformed into a standard shape first – usually the mean shape of the SSM. The appearance model is then created by performing a PCA on

the covariance matrix of textures. As with the profile models, normalization of the intensities is generally useful: This can be accomplished by adding an offset and by scaling to transform all gray-values to zero-mean and unit-variance [40], or by a non-linear procedure as described by Bosch et al. [17]. The latter method proved especially useful in images with a strongly non-Gaussian distribution as encountered e.g. in ultrasound images. As an alternative to working with intensities, Cootes et al. [40] propose storing gradient direction and strength, the latter mapped non-linearly. In an evaluation on face images, this method proved to be better than the normalized intensity. Scott et al. [206] use gradient orientation, corner and edge strength for the detection of vertebrae in dual energy X-ray images. For the analysis of colored face images, Stegmann and Larsen [222] employ HSV color space and model appearance as value (i.e. intensity), hue and edge (gradient magnitude).

Obviously, memory requirements have to be taken into account when using data from the entire inner region of the model: Even in 2D, the involved matrices can get fairly large, and for 3D volumes or time series the problem is much more acute. Nonetheless, complete region-based appearance models can be built for these cases by reducing the resolution of the employed texture, as several studies demonstrate [169, 11, 17]. Another option is to use only certain parts of the region, e.g. rectangular regions around specific feature points, as proposed by Cristinacce et al. [47]. In this scheme, all local regions are independently intensity-normalized and then concatenated into one feature vector. Still, the most efficient way of using region information is to extract specific features from the region of interest. As an extreme example, Freedman et al. [84] propose to model appearance by the gray-value distribution (i.e. a histogram) of all voxels inside the examined object. To be able to better discriminate between the modeled object and the background, a widely used enhancement is to model both inner and outer regions of the SSM. Below, several works in this direction are presented, which can all be used in the classical Active Shape Model framework (Sec. 2.6.2).

Broadhurst et al. [24] create histograms for inside and outside regions and map these to Euclidean space using the Earth mover's distance, where they can apply PCA to the data. They also evaluate different methods of how to best define the used regions (e.g. only use pixels within a certain distance from the boundary) and compare their method to a boundary-based profile approach. In a subsequent publication [23], the authors enhance their ap-

proach by weighting the influence of each pixel and introducing a-priori information about the expected variance. Van Ginneken et al. [254] model the inside and outside appearance around each landmark using a number of derivatives at different scales (also called the local jet [80]). An optimal feature selection picks the best set of features for each landmark. During search, these best sets are employed to estimate the inside probability for a number of pixels on a profile using a kNN-classifier. The method has been tested on X-ray and MRI images and delivered better results than the Mahalanobis distance on gray value profiles. Later, the approach was modified by Ordas et al. [179] to use Cartesian Differential Invariants instead of the local jet, making it invariant to orientation. Zhan and Shen [267] employ Gabor filter banks to extract features from 3D ultrasound images. The features extracted by two Gabor filters in orthogonal planes are forwarded to a kernel support vector machine that estimates the likelihood of a voxel belonging to prostate tissue or not.

Recently, Larsen et al. [145] presented the first approach to employing feature extraction to the Active Appearance Model framework (Sec. 2.6.3): They represent object texture by wavelets and wedgelets, thus not only reducing the dimensionality of texture vectors, but also reducing noise. Due to the inherent frequency separation, emphasis on edges can be incorporated without additional computational costs.

### 2.5.3 Clustering techniques

A common approach to building appearance models is to train one model for every landmark of the SSM. However, almost all of the local methods described above can benefit from clustering: In this case, several landmarks with similar boundary appearance are combined to train a shared appearance model. The obvious advantage is that clustered models are based on more training samples and thus offer improved generalization ability.

Brejl et al. [20] describe the first use of clustering for appearance models, employing the c-means algorithm to generate a user-specified number of $n$ clusters from all landmarks in all training images. During search, they compare the sampled features with all $n$ models and select the boundary fitting costs of the most similar one. To enable utilization of different models for different parts of the boundary, they suggest a manual definition of the respective border segments and storage of those models that are allowed for each one. Only the allowed models are then compared with the sampled features. Kaus et al. present a more practical solution in [127]: After clustering

all features into n classes with the k-means algorithm, each landmark is assigned to the cluster containing the largest number of training features from that point. During search, the features sampled at a certain landmark only need to be compared with the assigned cluster. Different appearance models for different boundary segments are thus supported automatically. Stough et al. [225] reach the same result with a different method: After the clustering process, they assign each landmark to the one cluster that returns the best accumulated fitting costs for all training features at that point. In their work, these fitting costs are calculated by the normalized correlation between the sample feature and a prototype generated for each cluster.

While the presented approaches cluster boundary appearance with respect to the feature values, Ho et al. [112] suggest a spatial clustering. Working with profile models, they define a profile scale-space and combine profiles hierarchically based on their neighborhood relation. In this case, the neighborhood relation is defined on a sphere and thus requires objects of spherical topology to work. The results are profiles that are blurred along the boundary, like in case of directional smoothing.

## 2.6 Search Algorithms

Due to the large size of the search space in 3D, most methods applied to locate an SSM in new image data use local search algorithms that require an initial estimate of the model pose. In the first subsection, several approaches for this initialization are reviewed, including some global search algorithms that deliver a complete solution for shape and pose. Subsequently, the popular Active Shape Models and Active Appearance Models with some of their variants are treated. In a next step, various alternative search algorithms are discussed, and finally methods for the refinement of detected shapes and the incorporation of user interaction are presented.

### 2.6.1 Initialization

The easiest solution to initializing an SSM is user interaction, as implemented e.g. in [128, 262, 193, 139, 201]. In general, it is sufficient to roughly align the position and rotation of the mean shape to the data, which can be accomplished in negligible time (less than half a minute). For cases requiring a more specific initialization, Hug et al. [117] propose to manually

specify a small number (usually three to four) of points that define a principal control polygon for the shape. In certain cases, these control points can also be detected automatically by using learned confidence regions.

As an alternative to manual interaction, other image processing techniques may be employed for initialization: Soler et al. [216] estimate the position of a liver model from histogram information extracted from the image, and Fripp et al. [87] perform an affine registration with an atlas to determine the starting position for an SSM of the knee cartilage. Brejl and Sonka [20] extend the Generalized Hough transform to incorporate shape variability and use this method successfully for 2D segmentation. However, the necessary accumulator array seems unfeasible for 3D since the number of array dimensions would increase from four to seven (if using the proposed similarity transformation).

Last but not least, there is the possibility of conducting a global search on the entire image. Due to the large search space and numerous local minima, this task is predestined for the use of evolutionary algorithms (EA). Already in the 1970s, Holland [114] developed one of the most popular variants of EA, the genetic algorithms: A large population of solutions (each one encoded as a binary chromosome) is initially spread across the entire search space and evaluated simultaneously. According to these results, the best set of chromosomes is selected for reproduction to produce the next generation of solutions. Mimicking biological evolution, there are mutation (random bit changes) and cross-over operators which influence the process. After several iterations/generations, the best-rated chromosome in the population is regarded as the final solution. Hill et al. [110] were the first to employ genetic algorithms for the model-based segmentation of echocardiogram images, optimizing 4 pose and 6 shape parameters (all encoded in one chromosome) of a custom-built model. They also presented an extension called *niches and species* to the algorithm in order to detect several candidate shapes at once. Subsequently [108], this approach was used in the automatic detection of PDMs with one extension: The mutation part was not conducted randomly, but by a small number of local search iterations. This method – termed ASM mutation – lead to significant improvements in both speed of convergence and accuracy of the final solution. Stegmann et al. [221] employed a similar approach to initializing an SSM, albeit without reproduction of solutions: They start with large initial population, run a few local AAM searches on each one and select the best set. This set is refined by an additional number of AAM searches, and finally the best solution is

used as initialization. Pitiot et al. [192] present a hybrid search method that combines a deformable template with an evolutionary algorithm. Several *families* (comparable to the niches and species by Hill et al. [110]) analyze different areas in the search space at the same time. Better fitting families are allocated more children to intensify the search in these areas.

An algorithm which is closely related to genetic algorithms is particle filtering, which has become popular among the computer vision community under the name of condensation, by Isard and Blake [120]. The main differences are that particle filtering does not have a cross-over operator and that the mutation is not implemented by bit changes, but by Gaussian noise. De Bruijne and Nielsen employed the algorithm for SSM search in [58] and subsequently also with an extension for multiple objects in [59].

### 2.6.2 Active Shape Model search

Since their introduction by Cootes et al. [42, 43], Active Shape Models (ASMs) have become one of the most popular model-based segmentation techniques in medical imaging. ASM is a local search algorithm based on a point distribution model; an instance of the model $\mathbf{y}$ in an image is defined by a similarity transform $\mathsf{T}$ and shape parameters $\mathbf{b}$:

$$\mathbf{y} = \mathsf{T}\,(\bar{\mathbf{x}} + \Phi\mathbf{b}) \tag{2.8}$$

where $\Phi = (\phi_1 \dots \phi_c)$ is the matrix of eigenvectors. >From an initial state, adjustments are calculated individually for each landmark by evaluating the fit of the appearance model at different positions along the normal vector to the surface. This leads to a vector of optimal displacements $\mathbf{dy_p}$. In a first step, the pose $\mathsf{T}$ of the model is adjusted by a Procrustes match of the model to $\mathbf{y} + \mathbf{dy_p}$, leading to a new transform $\mathsf{T}$ and new residual displacements $\mathbf{dy_s}$. In a second step, $\mathbf{dy_s}$ is transformed into model space and then projected into parameter space to give the optimal parameter updates:

$$\mathbf{db} = \mathsf{P}^\mathsf{T}\tilde{\mathsf{T}}^{-1}\,(\mathbf{dy_s}) \tag{2.9}$$

where $\tilde{\mathsf{T}}$ is equal to $\mathsf{T}$ but without the translational part. After updating $\mathbf{b}$ and applying appropriate parameter limits (see Sec. 2.3.2), an updated valid instance of the model is the result. These two steps are conducted iteratively, until a specified convergence criterion is hit, e.g. the maximum or average landmark movement is below a given threshold. The most detailed description of the algorithm can be found in a technical report by Cootes

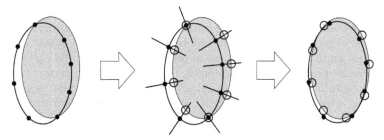

**Figure 2.8:** One iteration of an ASM search: At the beginning, the model (contour with landmarks) is located at the lower left of the true position (solid gray object). Local appearance models for all landmarks are evaluated at different positions perpendicular to the model surface. The best positions are shown as small circles in the center image. Finally, model parameters are updated to minimize the squared distances to the found best positions, bringing the model closer to the correct solution.

and Taylor [41]. Figure 2.8 shows a simple 2D example of the update procedure.

One of the first extensions to the basic ASM algorithm was the introduction of a coarse-to-fine search strategy in [44]: For this variant, the image data is organized as a multi-resolution pyramid and the SSM has separate appearance models for each level. The search starts at the coarsest level and switches to the next resolution when a predefined criterion is met, e.g. when the optimal displacement positions are located in the central part of the search profile for 95% of all landmarks. This procedure leads to a considerable increase in speed, robustness and quality of fit; it is commonly employed in all recent publications using ASMs. Another extension by Hill et al. [109] introduces correctional constraints for shape approximation: In both Procrustes matching and shape parameter calculation, the error term based on **dy** is split into two weighted parts, one normal to the surface and one tangential. By weighting the tangential part lower than the normal, landmarks can slide along the surface more easily. In experiments with 2D images this leads to faster convergence and better accuracy, for 3D images the algorithm is described but not evaluated.

The largest part of proposed modifications to the original ASM algorithm tries to improve the stability against outliers: The default least-squares approach is only optimal for a Gaussian distribution of residuals [7], and out-

liers in the appearance model match can disturb the search considerably, especially if they occur clustered. Duta and Sonka [71] propose detecting and correcting outliers by using the variance information from the PDM: The influence of each updated point position on the change of shape parameters is compared to the average point influence. If it is too large, the point is considered an outlier and corrected based on the position of its neighbors. Lekadir et al. [147] employ a shape metric based on the ratio of landmark distances to detect outliers. If a candidate point is located outside a trained confidence interval, a replacement point is suggested for further processing. In addition, detected outliers are stored and used to modify a weighting factor for the appearance model, effectively reducing the search space and preventing future outliers in that part of the boundary.

Instead of trying to identify and correct outliers, several works have tried to decrease their influence using the weighting of residuals $\mathbf{dy}$. Rogers and Graham [203] evaluate the use of M-estimators, image match and random sampling for this purpose: For M-estimators, the landmark weights depend on the size of the residuals; points with large residuals are weighted less than others, reducing their influence. For the image match method, the weights are set to the probability of fit for the local appearance model at the respective location. In random sampling, shape parameters are estimated based on a number of different random subsets of landmarks (i.e. using a binary weighting), which are combined afterwards. In a concluding evaluation, the random sampling was the most effective of these three methods. Li and Chutatape [150] suggest that pose and shape optimization are conducted twice: For the second run, weights are set according to the remaining residuals after the first optimization. If that failed to decrease the residual for a specific landmark below a given threshold, the relevant landmark is weighted down or not considered at all. Zhao at al. [270] combine values from the fit of the current appearance model, the stability of point positions during the last iteration and the stability of appearance model into one weight matrix. In an evaluation on face images, this procedure leads to more accurate results than those achieved without weighting.

Yet another approach to treat outliers is proposed by Nahed et al. [173]: Firstly, a number of candidate feature points are extracted from the image around the current model position. In a next step, a robust point matching algorithm which rejects outliers [92] is used to find the best-fitting model. A method which is not applicable to 3D but which is very efficient in 2D is to employ a minimum cost search for the boundary as proposed by Behiels et

al. [9]. In this approach, the difference of neighboring candidate positions (i.e. the shift perpendicular to the surface) is penalized and weighted with the fit of the appearance model, leading to an optimal solution with respect to the defined cost function.

### 2.6.3 Active Appearance Model search

Active Appearance Models (AAMs), introduced by Cootes et al. in [30], belong to the class of generative models, i.e. they can synthesize realistic images of the modeled data. This is made possible by storing the complete appearance (or texture) of the object, including its variations, in addition to the expected shape. However, AAMs are more than shape models with region-based features; they also feature a proprietary search method which differs completely from ASMs. Shape and appearance variation are combined into one linear system, allowing for shape $\mathbf{x}$ and appearance $\mathbf{g}$ to be described by a common parameter vector $\mathbf{b}$:

$$\begin{aligned} \mathbf{x} &= \bar{\mathbf{x}} + \Phi_s \mathbf{b} \\ \mathbf{g} &= \bar{\mathbf{g}} + \Phi_g \mathbf{b} \end{aligned} \tag{2.10}$$

where $\Phi_s$ and $\Phi_g$ are eigenvector matrices of the shape or gray-value model, respectively. An instance of an AAM in an image is thus defined by a similarity transformation $\mathsf{T}$ and the combined shape-appearance parameters $\mathbf{b}$ – below, both together are denoted as parameters $\mathbf{p}$. To evaluate the goodness of fit, the image texture is warped to the mean shape and normalized, resulting in $\mathbf{g_s}$. Using the modeled gray-value appearance $\mathbf{g_m} = \mathbf{g}$ from Eq. 2.10, the residuals are then given by $\mathbf{r}(\mathbf{p}) = \mathbf{g_s} - \mathbf{g_m}$, and the error by $E = \mathbf{r}^2$.

The key idea of AAM search is to assume a constant relationship between texture residuals $\mathbf{r}(\mathbf{p})$ and parameter updates $\mathbf{dp}$ over the entire search:

$$\mathbf{dp} = -R\mathbf{r}(\mathbf{p}) \tag{2.11}$$

The success of this optimization scheme largely depends on the derivative matrix R. In the first presentation of AAMs [30], R was computed using multivariate linear regression on a large number of simulated disturbances of the training images. Later, regression was replaced by numeric differentiation, claimed to be both faster and more reliable [32]. Donner et al. [68] point out a more practical advantage of the latter approach, i.e. it does not require the loading of all training images into memory at once for training.

AAMs quickly gained popularity in the image analysis community, and several modifications to the original scheme were proposed. A review of the early variants is given by Cootes and Kittipanya-ngam [33], who compare Shape AAMs [31] (which only update pose and shape by residuals, while texture is updated directly), compositional updating [5] (using thin-plate splines for the pose update) and Direct AAMs [116] (which predict shape by texture). More recent modifications include the work of Matthews and Baker [163], who suggest an inverse compositional warp update instead of the standard additive update and present an analytical derivation for a gradient descent search. Beichel et al. [10] partition the residuals $\mathbf{r}(\mathbf{p})$ into different modes using the mean-shift algorithm. During search, they match the image to all different combinations of modes and calculate parameter updates for every single one. For each iteration they accept the combination leading to the best result of the objective function, thus rejecting up to 50% of outliers. Donner et al. [68] employ canonical correlation analysis to calculate the derivative matrix R. This method provides more accurate estimates for parameter updates than the standard numeric differentiation, resulting in a search that is up to four times faster. In addition, it requires fewer examples in the training phase, thus also speeding up the model construction considerably.

Although AAMs are mainly described for 2D (a prominent application is face recognition), the method itself is by no means limited in dimension. Mitchell et al. [169] presented the first true 3D model, using volumetric textures to represent appearance. More 3D medical applications are described in Sec. 2.7. A good starting point to experiment with AAMs is the open source software FAME by Stegmann et al. [220] – although it currently only supports 2D models. As with ASMs, the most detailed description of the basic algorithm is given in the technical report by Cootes and Taylor [41]. Figure 2.9 shows a simple 2D example of the update procedure.

### 2.6.4 Other algorithms with strict shape constraints

Though ASM and AAM are the most frequently employed constrained search algorithms, there exist several other possibilities to fit an SSM to new data. After initialization of the model, standard optimization techniques can be used to directly optimize the shape parameters. Successfully employed algorithms include the Nelder-Mead simplex approach (used by Heinze et al. [104] and Tang and Ellis [235]), the Quasi-Newton method (used by Haslam et al. [98] and Székely et al. [233]), the conjugate gradient (CG) algo-

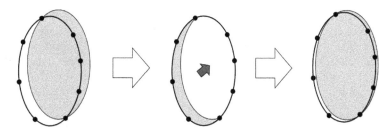

**Figure 2.9:** One iteration of an AAM search: Initially, the model (contour with landmarks) is located at the lower left of the true position (solid gray object). The texture beneath the model is sampled and compared to the region-based appearance model. The corresponding residuals are shown in the center image and suggest a move of the model to the upper right – this information is learned during training and encoded in matrix R. The resulting parameter update does indeed bring the model closer to the correct solution.

rithm (used by Staib and Duncan [219] and Lötjönen et al. [160]) and gradient descent optimization (used by Freedman et al. [84] and Nain et al. [174]). In general though, these methods are slower than the approaches presented above: Haslam et al. [98] report a runtime for the Quasi-Newtonian optimizer that is 50 times longer than ASM. Therefore, the standard optimization techniques are mainly used in cases where ASM is not applicable, either because the SSM uses a different shape representation (no PDM), or because the appearance model does not allow the individual evaluation of fit for each landmark.

For volumetric shape models, Rueckert et al. [204] present a method called *statistical deformation models*. Here, the statistical analysis is not conducted by using point coordinates, but rather by using volumetric deformation fields between a mean image (the atlas) and training samples. The results are used to constrain the B-splines registration of the atlas to new images, reducing the search space considerably.

Klim et al. [133] present a mixture of the described ASM and AAM methods: They use a standard PDM with edge-based appearance models for all landmarks, which determine the individual best fits along the respective normal vectors. But instead of using the ASM procedure to update parameters, they employ a regression matrix as in AAM optimization. The method is only evaluated for 2D (with better performance than ASM on hand x-rays), but could also be implemented for the 3D case.

### 2.6.5 Algorithms with relaxed shape constraints

In the preceding sections (Secs. 2.6.1–2.6.4), algorithms which strictly adhere to the underlying SSM have been discussed. Below, various methods to relax the hard shape constraints and to allow for additional flexibility during search are described.

One approach to solving this problem is to run a normal SSM until convergence and to include an additional refinement step afterwards. The rationale behind this is that the model surface should be close enough to the real contour at that stage to be attracted with edge-based features. Shang and Dossel [207] simply search for the best fit of each individual vertex within a confined local neighborhood, guided by the local appearance models. However, in the absence of shape constraints, some kind of regularization is generally required to deal with noise and image clutter. To this end, Cootes and Taylor [37] examine the candidate positions suggested by the individual local appearance models and conduct a pruned tree search to determine the subset of points that best matches the current shape model. Li and Reinhardt [149] employ a slice-wise contour refinement for the segmented volume: In each slice, the 2D contour is adjusted and regularized by a snake, which draws its external energy from the local appearance models. Pekar et al. [186] utilize a freely deformable triangular mesh that is initialized with the converged SSM and regularized by its internal smoothness constraints.

Another class of methods introduces additional flexibility already from the start of the search: Such approaches are typically based on a deformable mesh that bases its internal energies on the discrepancy to the closest allowed shape model. Weese et al. [262] use the differences in corresponding edge lengths between mesh and model for this purpose and employ a conjugate gradient algorithm to optimize all point positions. Shen et al. [210] use the difference between learned attribute vectors (characterizing the geometric structure of the model) and the current mesh as basis for internal energy. They employ local affine transformations, modulated by a Gaussian envelop function, to adjust the deformable model. Due to the ability to weight different parts of the model differently during search, this algorithm is termed *Adaptive Focus Deformable Shape Model* (AFDSM). Tsagaan et al. [245] model shape variation based on local curvature feature vectors, which are used to calculate covariance matrices during training. The internal energy for the search is then based on the Mahalanobis distances from the features of the current mesh to the stored data. For the m-rep shape

representation by Pizer et al. [193], a special deformation scheme has been developed: In a hierarchical procedure, the entire SSM is first fitted globally, then individual subfigures and subsequently the medial atoms are adjusted (all using a conjugate gradient optimizer). The last step is a refinement of the boundary vertices along the corresponding normal vectors.

### 2.6.6 Incorporation of user interaction

A topic which has received relatively little attention until now is that of incorporation of user interaction into SSM search algorithms. In case of a failure of automatic segmentation, the user should be able to correct the result by moving a limited number of incorrectly placed landmarks to their true positions. The most elegant solution to this problem is presented by Cootes and Taylor [39]: They define a probabilistic framework for AAMs, in which the error function is enhanced to include priors on parameters and point positions. In this way, the additional data is integrated seamlessly into the segmentation process. Neumann and Lorenz [175], working with an ASM-like search algorithm, suggest adding a new error term to the least-squares procedure which fits model points to candidate locations in each iteration. The resulting linear system of equations can be solved analytically for 2D shapes, but for 3D an iterative procedure is required. Van Ginneken et al. [253] propose running the standard ASM shape parameter update repeatedly: Every time, landmarks that have been corrected by the user are set to their specified positions again, until the shape model converges towards these positions. An evaluation in the same paper reveals that too many manually corrected landmarks actually result in a deterioration of the performance of the SSM, because the deformation becomes too restricted.

## 2.7 Applications

In this section, applications of 3D SSMs for medical image analysis are presented. The focus is on the medical application, i.e. only those papers are listed which state a real-world problem solvable with the approach. Studies where a shape model is built only to demonstrate the feasibility of the modeling approach will not be considered.

| Authors | Object(s) of interest | Modality | Correspondences | Appearance | Search |
|---|---|---|---|---|---|
| | | | Bone structures | | |
| Pekar et al. [186] | Vertebrae | CT | Mesh-to-mesh | G-Profile (Untr) | Deformable |
| Davatzikos et al. [50] | Spine | MRI | Mesh-to-volume | G-Profile (Untr) | AFDSM |
| Heinze et al. [104] | Knee joint | CT | Point matching | Profile (Expl) | ICP + Simplex PF |
| Fripp et al. [88] | Knee bones | MRI | Optimization | ? | ASM |
| Josephson et al. [123] | Knee (femur) | MRI | Point matching | I-Profile (Mah) | ASM |
| Tang and Ellis [235] | Femur | Multi X-Ray | Point matching | G-Profile (Cor) | Simplex PF |
| Lamecker et al. [139] | Pelvic bone | CT | Man + Param | Profile (Expl) | ASM |
| | | | Brain structures | | |
| Székely et al. [233] | Deep brain structures | MRI | SPHARM | G-Profile (Untr) | Quasi-Newton PF |
| Staib and Duncan[219] | Caudate nucleus | MRI | Parameterization | G-Profile (Untr) | CG PF |
| Kelemen et al. [128] | Caudate nucleus | MRI | SPHARM | I-Profile (Mah) | ASM-like |
| Nain et al. [174] | Caudate, hippocampus | MRI | Parameterization | I-Region | GD PF |
| Shenton et al. [213] | Hippocampus | MRI | SPHARM | I-Profile (Mah) | ASM-like |
| Duchesne et al. [70] | Hippocampus | MRI | Volume-to-volume | NI-Region (Res) | AAM-like |
| Pizer et al. [193] | Hippocampus | MRI | Mesh-to-volume | NG-Profile (Cor) | m-rep |
| Klemencic et al. [132] | Hippocampus | MRI | Volume-to.volume | NI-Region (Res) | AAM-like |
| Shen et al. [210, 211] | Deep brain structures | MRI | Mesh-to-volume | G-Profile (Untr) | AFDSM |
| Bailleul et al. [4] | Deep brain structures | MRI | Optimization | Profile (Expl) | ASM |
| Zhao et al. [271] | Deep brain structures | MRI | Mesh-to-volume | Not specified | partitioned ASM |
| Caunce and Taylor [27] | Cortical sulci | MRI | Mesh-to-mesh | I-Profile (Mah) | ASM |
| Tao et al. [237] | Cortical sulci | MRI | Parameterization | F-Region (Mah) | Spherical warps |
| Lao et al. [141] | Cortical surface | MRI | Mesh-to-volume | G-Profile (Untr) | AFDSM |
| Josephson et al.[123] | Cortical surface | SPECT | Point matching | I-Profile (Mah) | ASM |
| | | | Cardiac structures | | |
| Staib and Duncan [219] | Left ventricle | MRI | Parameterization | G-Profile (Untr) | CG PF |
| Mitchell et al. [169] | Left ventricle | MRI | Parameterization | NI-Region (Res) | AAM |
| Lapp et al. [142] | Ventricles, myocardium | MRI + CT | Volume-to-volume | NI-Region (Res) | AAM |
| Kaus et al. [127] | Left ventricle | MRI | Mesh-to-volume | Profile (Expl) | Deformable |
| van Assen et al. [251] | Left ventricle | MSCT | Arc-length | I-Profile (Class) | ASM |
| Fritz et al. [90] | Left ventricle | MSCT | Parameterization | I-Profile (Mah) | ASM |
| Stegmann and Pedersen [223] | Left ventricle | dyn. MRI | Arc-length | NI-Region (Res) | AAM |
| Lötjönen et al. [160] | Heart | MRI | Volume-to-volume | I-Region (NMI) | CG PF and others |
| Shang and Dossel [207] | Left ventricle | MRI | Mesh-to-volume | G-Profile (Untr) | ASM + Refinement |
| Fritz et al. [89] | Cardiac chambers | MSCT | Mesh-to-mesh | Profile (Expl) | ASM |
| Lorenz and von Berg [158] | Heart (incl. vessels) | MSCT | Mesh-to-volume | Profile (Expl) | Deformable |
| van Assen et al. [252] | Left ventricle | Sparse MRI | Volume-to-volume | I-Profile (Class) | sparse ASM |
| Zambal et al. [266] | Left ventricle | MRI | Parameterization | NI-Region (Res) | combined 2D AAMs |
| Nahed et al. [173] | Right ventricle | MRI | Optimization | G-Profile (Untr) | Point matching |
| Tölli et al. [244] | Heart | MRI | Volume-to-volume | var. Profiles | var. PF & Global |
| | | | Soft tissue structures in the abdominal and pelvic area | | |
| Dickens et al. [67] | Kidney | Synthetic | Manual | I-Profile (Mah) | ASM |
| Tsagaan et al. [245] | Kidney | CT | Manual | G-Profile (Untr) | Deformable |
| Pizer et al. [193] | Kidney | CT | Mesh-to-volume | NI-Profile (Cor) | m-rep |
| Stough et al. [225], Rao et al. [201] | Kidney | CT | Mesh-to-volume | cl.NI-Profile (Cor) | m-rep |
| Beichel et al. [11] | Diaphragm dome | CT | Manual | NI-Region (Res) | combined 2D AAMs |
| Lamecker et al. [138, 137] | Liver | CT | Man + Param | I-Profile (Expl) | ASM |
| Lim and Ho [155] | Liver | CT | Mesh-to-mesh | F-Profile (Mah) | ASM |
| Pekar et al. [187] | Bladder, rectum, fem.h. | CT | Mesh-to-volume | Profile (Expl) | Deformable |
| Zhan and Shen [267] | Prostate | 3D-US | Mesh-to-volume | F-Region (Class) | AFDSM |
| Hodge et al. [113] | Prostate | US | Optimization | Not specified | ASM |
| de Bruijne et al. [61] | Aortic aneurysms | CT | Parameterization | I-Profile (Class) | ASM |
| de Bruijne et al. [62] | Aortic aneurysms | CT | Parameterization | I-Profile (Class) | combined 2D ASMs |

**Table 2.1:** 3D segmentation tasks solved with statistical shape models. Refer to the text for a description of abbreviations (Sec. 2.7.1).

### 2.7.1 Segmentation

According to this survey, 3D segmentation – i.e. the analysis and labeling of volumetric images – is the major application of statistical shape models. With the arrival of automatic landmarking methods, this field has experienced an enormous boost, and publication numbers continue to rise. SSMs have been used for the segmentation of a variety of structures in the human body. To provide the reader with an overview, all publications are sorted in Table 2.1, grouped by the analyzed body parts: Bone structures, brain structures, cardiac structures and soft tissue structures in the abdominal and pelvic area. Each entry in the table contains information about the modeled object of interest, the image modality, and the techniques used for the work. Specifically, the method used to acquire the required point correspondences is listed as:

- Point matching, Mesh-to-mesh: see Sec. 2.4.1

- Mesh-to-volume: see Sec. 2.4.2

- Volume-to-volume: see Sec. 2.4.3

- Arc-length, SPHARM, Parameterization: see Sec. 2.4.4

- Optimization: see Sec. 2.4.5

- Manual: pure manual landmarking

- Man + X: manual landmarking for a limited set of points, followed by an automatic propagation method

The employed appearance model is categorized as *Profile* (Sec. 2.5.1) or *Region* (Sec. 2.5.2). If applicable, the type of feature used is given as:

- I, NI: (Normalized) intensity

- G, NG: (Normalized) gradient

- F: extracted features like wavelet coefficients etc.

A *cl.* in front indicates that the appearance model is clustered. The selection strategy or rating method for the fit of an appearance model at a new position is given at the end in parenthesis. Possible values are:

- Untr: Untrained model, usually search for the strongest gradient etc.

- Expl: Explicit rules defining the best appearance

- Mah: Mahalanobis distance to Gaussian appearance model

- Cor: Correlation to one or several learned templates

- Class: Classification into foreground/background or edge/non-edge

- Res: Residuals to Gaussian appearance model, used for AAMs

Finally, the search algorithm is listed as:

- ASM: Active Shape Model, see Sec. 2.6.2

- AAM: Active Appearance Model, see Sec. 2.6.3

- PF: Parameter fitting by Nelder-Mead Simplex, Quasi-Newton, or conjugate gradient (CG) optimization, see Sec. 2.6.4

- Deformable, AFDSM, m-rep: Algorithms based on deformable models with extended variability, see Sec. 2.6.5

### 2.7.2 Other applications

In addition to segmentation, SSMs are employed to a variety of other applications in medical image analysis. One common task is that of shape analysis, i.e. the correlation of the shape of certain structures to patient-specific attributes in clinical studies. In the simplest case, this is accomplished by classifying the shape parameter vector of the object of interest into one of several groups. Another common task is the extrapolation of shapes from sparse 3D data to detailed representation, as required for some intra-operative navigation scenarios. Hawkes et al. [99] have published a discussion paper about models in image-guided interventions, which closer reviews some works in that area. An overview of some applications other than segmentation is given in Table. 2.2. The terms used for correspondences are the same as in Table. 2.1, refer to Sec. 2.7.1 for details.

| Authors | Object(s) of interest | Correspondences | Application |
|---|---|---|---|
| | | Shape analysis | |
| Paulsen et al. [184, 185] | Ear canal | Mesh-to-mesh | Correlation to gender |
| Styner at al. [226, 227] | Hippocampus | SPHARM | Correlation to schizophrenia |
| Davies et al. [54] | Hippocampus | Optimization | Correlation to schizophrenia |
| Csernansky et al. [48] | Thalamus | Volume-to-volume | Correlation to schizophrenia |
| Kim et al. [130] | Hippocampus | Mesh-to-volume | Correlation to schizophrenia |
| Bansal et al. [6] | Hippocampus, amygdala | Volume-to-volume | Correlation to attention deficit / hyperactivity disorder |
| Thompson et al. [241] | Hippocampus, ventricles | Man + Param | Correlation to Alzheimer disease |
| Styner at al. [226] | Brain ventricles | SPHARM | Correlation to twins |
| Ferrarini et al. [75] | Brain ventricles | Mesh-to-mesh | Correlation to aging |
| Wang et al. [260] | Cortical surface | Mesh-to-mesh | Correlation to neurologic and psychiatric disorders |
| | | Shape extrapolation | |
| Fleute et al. [77] | Femur | Mesh-to-mesh | Extrapolate geometry from sparse 3D data for surgery |
| Chan et al. [28] | Femur | Volume-to-volume | Extrapolate geometry from sparse 3D data for surgery |
| Zheng et al. [273], Rajamani et al. [199] | Femoral heads | Optimization | Extrapolate geometry from sparse 3D data for surgery |
| | | Other applications | |
| Subsol et al. [230] | Crest lines on skull | Mesh-to-mesh | Assess mandible deformation under craniofacial disease |
| Andresen et al. [2] | Mandible | Mesh-to-mesh | Model mandible growth |
| Blackall et al. [13] | Liver | Volume-to-volume | Model deformation caused by breathing |
| Rueckert et al. [204] | Brain | Volume-to-volume | Register landmarks to new subjects |
| Lee et al. [146] | Levator ani | Optimization | Optimal scan planning |
| Deligianni et al. [64] | Bronchial tree | Feature points | Model breathing motion for bronchoscopy simulation |
| Sierra et al. [214] | Uterus | Man+Subdivision | Generate variable scenes for surgery simulator |

**Table 2.2:** 3D statistical shape models built for other medical applications (non-segmentation).

# 3 Shape Model Construction

*Without geometry, life is pointless.*

— *Anonymous*

In this chapter, methods developed to automatically generate statistical shape models for medical 3D data are illustrated. For maximum flexibility and ease of use, models are based on a representation by landmarks. Therefore, the major challenge in model construction is the location of required point correspondences on training data. For this purpose, a population-based optimization approach is presented, which has a number of advantages over existing techniques.

Section 3.1 briefly describes the procedure to generate training surfaces from labeled image volumes. Subsequently, a parameterization method to map these surfaces to the unit sphere is presented in Sec. 3.2. The obtained parameterizations are the basis for the following correspondence modification, which is driven by a gradient-based minimization scheme, as explained in Sec. 3.3. In Sec. 3.4, this approach is extended by a landmark reconfiguration procedure that results in more accurate shape models. Finally, the chapter concludes with the presentation of new performance measures to evaluate the quality of models produced.

## 3.1 Generation of training meshes

There exist several well established methods to convert labeled volumetric data (i.e. segmentations) to surfaces, the most popular one being the Marching Cubes algorithm by Lorensen and Cline [156]. However, since the resulting surfaces are input to a population-based optimization approach (as presented in Sec. 3.3), there are certain requirements that have to be fulfilled. Most importantly, surfaces must be of genus zero topology (i.e. without holes and self-intersections) to enable the generation of parameterizations in the next step. Secondly, they should also be reasonably smooth,

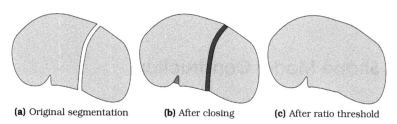

**(a)** Original segmentation **(b)** After closing **(c)** After ratio threshold

**Figure 3.1:** A 2D example for the intelligent closing method. The original segmentation (a) features a tunnel that has to be closed and a smaller gap which should remain as it is. After a normal closing operation (b), both tunnel (blue) and gap (red) are filled. The tunnel has about twice as many voxels adjacent to the background as the gap, but a much larger volume. Thus, the ratio of voxels adjacent to the background is lower for the tunnel. Employing thresholding with this criterion, the tunnel closing is kept, but the gap filling is rejected, resulting in the final processed segmentation (c).

as this leads to a faster convergence of correspondence optimization, and in any case, details too fine cannot be captured by the statistical model.

To fulfill these requirements, the following processing pipeline to generate training meshes is employed: The first step runs a 3x3x3 median filter on the segmented volume to remove label inconsistencies, especially between neighboring slices. As most training data is manually segmented in a slice-by-slice-fashion, these inconsistencies appear quite frequently. The following step, though optional, consists of a morphological closing operation. It is required for objects of interest which are transversed by large vessels that are often not unlabeled, thus leaving tunnels throughout segmented objects. To prevent an over-smoothing effect on the outer surface, newly added components are sorted according to their ratio of voxels adjacent to background areas. Only components where this ratio is below a given threshold are retained (Fig. 3.1). Subsequently, the resulting segmentation (usually labeled value 1) is set to a value of 100 and smoothed by Gaussian low-pass filtering. This step prevents the stairs effect on anisotropically spaced data when the Marching Cubes algorithm is run later on and leads to smoother surfaces. The followin step is called *island removal*. In some segmentations, there exist small labeled regions aside from the object of interest which must be deleted. This is accomplished using a connected component analysis and by retaining the largest object. The final prepro-

cessing step is to fill potential holes inside the remaining object. Upon completion, the training mesh is generated by the Marching Cubes algorithm, run with a threshold of 50 (half the value of the label field before the Gaussian filtering). The resulting meshes can directly be used as an input for the parameterization step.

## 3.2 Mesh parameterization

To define an initial set of correspondences and a means of manipulating them efficiently, a convenient base domain for landmarks on the training shapes is required. For closed 2D objects, the natural choice for this base domain is the arc-length position on the contour. Choosing an arbitrary starting point and normalizing the total arc-length to 1, all positions on the contour (i.e. all potential landmark positions) can be described by a single parameter $p \in [0..1]$.

For closed 3D objects, the suitable base domain depends on the genus of the object, which determines how many holes the surface features. In order to minimize complexity for parameterization of 3D shapes, the discussion is restricted to closed two-manifolds of genus zero. Objects of this class are topologically equivalent to a sphere and comprise most shapes encountered in medical imaging, e.g. liver, kidneys and lungs. The task is to find a homeomorphic mapping which assigns every point on the surface of the mesh a unique position on the unit sphere, described by two parameters longitude $\theta \in [0..2\pi]$ and latitude $\phi \in [0..\pi]$. Formally, a parameterization function $\Omega$ is assigned to each training mesh of the shape model.

**Definition 1** *Each training sample for the SSM is represented as a triangulated mesh* $K = (\mathcal{V}, \mathcal{E})$ *with vertices* $u, v \in \mathcal{V}$ *and edges* $[u, v] \in \mathcal{E}$. *The vertex positions are specified by* $\mathbf{f} : \mathcal{V} \rightarrow R^3$, *an embedding function defined on the vertices of* K. *A second function* $\Omega : \mathcal{V} \rightarrow R^3$ *specifies the coordinates as mapped on the unit sphere,* $\forall v \in \mathcal{V} : |\Omega(v)| = 1$.

The mapping of an arbitrary shape to a sphere inevitably introduces some distortion. There are a number of different approaches which attempt to minimize this distortion, typically preserving either local angles or facet areas while trying to minimize distortions in the other. [1] For an initial parameterization, the current state of the art optimization by Davies et al. [55] uses

---

[1]An overview of recent work on this topic can be found in the survey by Floater and Hormann [79].

diffusion mapping, a simplified version of a method described by Brechbühler et al. [19] which is neither angle- nor area-preserving.

Due to the employed optimization strategy (Sec. 3.3), focus in this work lies on preserving angles: Moving neighboring points on the parameterization sphere in a specific direction, corresponding landmarks on the training shape should also move in a coherent direction. This behavior is guaranteed by conformal mapping functions, transformations that preserve local angles.

### 3.2.1 Creating a conformal mapping

To create a conformal parameterization, a variational method described by Gu et al. [96] and Wang et al. [259] is employed. The variational method uses a gradient descent optimization to minimize the string energy $E(K, \Omega)$, which is defined as the weighted sum over all edge lengths in the mesh:

$$E(K, \Omega) = \sum_{[u,v] \in \mathcal{E}} k_{u,v} |\Omega(v) - \Omega(u)| \tag{3.1}$$

with $k_{u,v}$ representing individual edge weights. When all edge weights are set to 1, this approach yields the barycentric mapping, where each vertex is positioned at the center of its neighbors – this is also known as *Tutte mapping*. A conformal mapping can be obtained by using edge weights that depend on opposing angles $\alpha, \beta$ of an edge $[u, v]$ as in:

$$k_{u,v} = \frac{1}{2} (\cot \alpha + \cot \beta) \tag{3.2}$$

Figure 3.2 demonstrates the location of these angles in an example constellation. Using the denotations from Fig. 3.2, the cotangens for $\alpha$ is calculated by:

$$\cot \alpha = \frac{(\mathbf{f}(u) - \mathbf{f}(a)) \cdot (\mathbf{f}(v) - \mathbf{f}(a))}{(\mathbf{f}(u) - \mathbf{f}(a)) \times (\mathbf{f}(v) - \mathbf{f}(a))} \tag{3.3}$$

The calculation of the cotangens for $\beta$ works equivalently.

Gu and Wang suggest to start minimization of the string energy from a Gauss map, where $\Omega(v)$ is initialized with the normal vector of $v$ in the original mesh defined by $\mathbf{f}(v)$. A first optimization is run with all $k_{u,v} = 1$ to generate a barycentric mapping. Following convergence, edge weights are set to the values given by Eq. 3.2 and a second optimization yields the conformal mapping. Both optimizations are based on the piecewise Laplacian

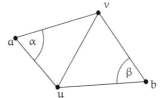

**Figure 3.2:** Edge $[u, v]$ with opposing angles $\alpha$ and $\beta$ in a triangular mesh.

$\nabla^2 \Omega$ of the mesh, which is calculated for each $u \in V$ by:

$$\nabla^2 \Omega(u) = \sum_{[u,v] \in \mathcal{E}} k_{u,v} \left( \Omega(v) - \Omega(u) \right) \tag{3.4}$$

$\nabla^2 \Omega$ can be separated into a normal and a tangential component. The normal component $\nabla^2 \Omega^{\perp}$ is given by:

$$(\nabla^2 \Omega(u))^{\perp} = \left( \nabla^2 \Omega(u) \cdot \mathbf{n}(\Omega(u)) \right) \cdot \mathbf{n}(\Omega(u)) \tag{3.5}$$

with $\mathbf{n}(\Omega(u))$ as the normal vector of $u$ in the parameterization. If the piecewise Laplacian consists only of this normal component, i.e. $\nabla^2 \Omega = \nabla^2 \Omega^{\perp}$, then $\Omega$ minimizes the string energy and is called a *harmonic* function.

Optimization of the string energy is implemented by a gradient descent approach that iteratively moves all vertices in the direction of the tangential component of $\nabla^2 \Omega$. The tangential component is also called absolute derivative and can be calculated by:

$$D\Omega(u) = \nabla^2 \Omega(u) - (\nabla^2 \Omega(u))^{\perp} \tag{3.6}$$

During the optimization process, all vertices must constantly be projected back onto the sphere by $\Omega(u) = \Omega'(u)/|\Omega'(u)|$. To prevent a collapse of all vertices to the same position, a centering step ensures that $\sum_{u \in V} \Omega(u) = 0$. The complete algorithm is shown in Fig. 3.3. To produce the barycentric mapping, a stepSize of $10^{-1}$ was utilized and convergence criterion $\epsilon$ was set to $10^{-4}$. For the subsequent conformal mapping, stepSize $= 10^{-2}$ and $\epsilon = 5 \cdot 10^{-5}$ were used.

### 3.2.2 Efficient landmark mapping

With an initial parameterization $\Omega_i$ for each training sample $i$, the necessary point correspondences can be acquired by mapping a set of spherical

---

**Algorithm 3.2.1:** MINIMIZESTRINGENERGY()

$energy \leftarrow$ GETSTRINGENERGY()
**repeat**
  **for each** $u \in \mathcal{V}$
    **do** $d_u \leftarrow$ GETABSOLUTEDERIVATIVE($u$)
  $center \leftarrow 0$
  **for each** $u \in \mathcal{V}$
    **do** $\begin{cases} \Omega(u) \leftarrow \Omega(u) + d_u \cdot stepSize \\ center \leftarrow center + \Omega(u)/|\mathcal{V}| \end{cases}$
  **for each** $u \in \mathcal{V}$
    **do** $\begin{cases} \Omega(u) \leftarrow \Omega(u) - center \\ \Omega(u) \leftarrow \Omega(u)/|\Omega(u)| \end{cases}$
  $newEnergy \leftarrow$ GETSTRINGENERGY()
  $\delta \leftarrow energy - newEnergy$
  $energy \leftarrow newEnergy$
**until** $(\delta < \epsilon)$

---

**Figure 3.3:** Pseudocode to minimize the string energy of a mesh.

coordinates to each shape. This set of spherical coordinates, in the following called landmark prototypes $\Psi$, is created by subdividing the icosahedron (with 12 vertices the largest of the Platonic solids) until the desired number of landmarks is reached. In practice, mostly three or four levels of subdivision are used, resulting in 642, respective 2562, equally distributed points on the sphere. After each level of subdivision, all newly inserted points have to be remapped to the sphere to comply with $|\Omega(v)| = 1$.

In order to obtain the 3D position on a training sample for a given landmark $\gamma \in \Psi$, it is necessary to find the intersection between a landmark-specific ray and the corresponding parameterization mesh. The ray begins at the origin of the sphere and is oriented towards the spherical coordinates of the landmark $(\theta_\gamma, \phi_\gamma)$. In general, it will not pass a vertex of the parameterization mesh, but one of the constituting triangles. To test a triangle for intersection, a method described by Möller and Trumbore [170] is employed, which conveniently produces the barycentric coordinates of the intersection point. Using these coordinates, which describe the relative position within the triangle, on the corresponding triangle in the training

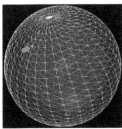 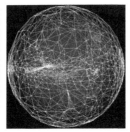 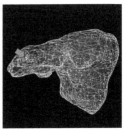

**(a)** Landmark on prototype **(b)** Ray through parameteri-    **(c)** Mapped landmark
                               zation

**Figure 3.4:** Landmark mapping from prototypes $\Psi$ to mesh. The landmark $\gamma$ (red arrow) is defined in a spherical coordinate system (a). The ray from the origin of the sphere through these coordinates intersects with exactly one triangle of the given parameterization mesh (b). The corresponding triangle of the training mesh defines the area where $\gamma$ will be mapped to, the exact location is determined by using barycentric coordinates inside the triangle.

mesh yields the final landmark position. The whole mapping process is visualized in Fig. 3.4 for an example of the liver.

During correspondence optimization (Sec. 3.3), parameterizations are constantly modified, which requires a frequent recalculation of mapped landmark positions. Since mapping landmarks is the most computationally expensive part of the model-building process, an intelligent search strategy of ordering the triangles according to the likelihood of ray intersection speeds up the algorithm considerably. Intersected triangle indices for each landmark are cached together with the barycentric coordinates of the intersection point. In the case of a cache miss, neighboring triangles are given priority when searching for the ray intersection. Figure 3.5 shows some pseudocode for the employed cache system.

## 3.3 Correspondence optimization

Although the initial correspondences[2] allow constructing an SSM, the resulting model is generally far from optimal. To improve the model by an optimization approach, the following components are required: A cost func-

---

[2]As described in Sec. 3.2, initial correspondences are defined by the locations the spherical landmark prototypes $\Psi$ get mapped to on different training shapes.

---

**Algorithm 3.2.2:** MAPLANDMARKPOINT(pntId)

**local** faceId, pos, hit
faceId ← cachedId$_\mathrm{pntId}$
**if not** FACEMODIFIED(faceId)
  **then return** (cachedPos$_\mathrm{pntId}$)
hit ← COORDINATESINFACE(pntId, faceId, pos)
**if not** hit
  **then** $\Biggl\{$   **for each** nbId ∈ $\mathcal{N}$(faceId)
          **do** $\Biggl\{$   hit ← COORDINATESINFACE(pntId, nbId, pos)
             **if** hit
                **then** $\Bigl\{$   faceId ← nbId
                         **exit**
**if not** hit
  **then** $\Biggl\{$   faceList ← SORTFACESBYDISTANCE(pntId)
          **for each** faceId ∈ faceList
          **do** $\Biggl\{$   hit ← COORDINATESINFACE(pntId, nbId, pos)
             **if** hit
               **then exit**
cachedId$_\mathrm{pntId}$ ← faceId
cachedPos$_\mathrm{pntId}$ ← pos
**return** (pos)

---

**Figure 3.5:** Pseudocode for the cache system to map a landmark from sphere to mesh. The method FACEMODIFIED(faceId) returns **true** if the indexed triangle has been modified since the last access, resulting in cache invalidity. The method COORDINATESINFACE(pntId, faceId, pos) tests the triangle indexed by faceId for intersection with a ray from the origin to the landmark coordinates given by pntId. If the ray hits the triangle, the method returns **true** and stores the resulting barycentric coordinates in pos. $\mathcal{N}$(faceId) is the set of neighboring faces for faceId, and SORTFACESBYDISTANCE(pntId) generates a list of all faces in the parameterization with ascending distance from the given landmark.

tion that describes the quality of the statistical model, a method to modify the existing correspondences and an efficient optimizer. In the following subsections, these three steps are presented in further detail.

### 3.3.1 Cost function

The cost function employed in this work is based on the Minimum Description Length (MDL) approach developed by Davies [52]. MDL has a sound theoretical foundation and has been shown to generate excellent correspondences (as described in Sec. 2.4.5). MDL weighs upon the premise that the simpler an SSM is, the better. This is in accordance with Occam's Razor and other strategies that strive for the simplest solution. The special property of an MDL approach is that it formalizes this strategy mathematically and finally presents a complete solution which is computable in reasonable time. The definition of *simple* is taken from Information Theory and means compact (or short) message. The SSM is used to encode the training samples, i.e. coordinates of different landmarks, in an information theoretic message. The shorter the resulting message, the more compact the model. In the following, the mathematics for the derivation of the cost function are briefly resumed.

**The encoding model**

Each training sample i, consisting of $n_l$ landmarks, is represented by an $(n_l d)$-dimensional vector $\mathbf{x}_i$. As stated in Eq. 2.4, this vector can be calculated given the principal modes of variation of the SSM:

$$\mathbf{x}^{(i)} = \bar{\mathbf{x}} + \sum_{m=1}^{n_s-1} b_m^{(i)} \phi_m \tag{3.7}$$

Thus, if the mean shape $\bar{\mathbf{x}}$ and the eigenvectors $\phi_m$ are known, it is sufficient to transmit the coefficients $b_m^{(i)}$ to recover the training samples. These define the position of the training sample in shape space and can be expressed as an $(n_s - 1)$-dimensional vector $\mathbf{b}^{(i)} = (b_1^{(i)} b_2^{(i)} \ldots b_{n_s-1}^{(i)})^T$. From the original data and the matrix of eigenvectors $\Phi$, this vector is calculated by:

$$\mathbf{b}^{(i)} = \Phi^T(\mathbf{x}^{(i)} - \bar{\mathbf{x}}) \tag{3.8}$$

Since it is assumed that coordinates in shape space follow a normal distribution with zero mean, the probability density function for a certain coeffi-

cient $b_m$ is defined by a Gaussian model with the standard deviation $\sigma_m$ as only parameter:

$$p(b_m, \sigma_m) = \frac{1}{\sqrt{2\pi\sigma_m^2}} \exp\left(-\frac{b_m^2}{2\sigma_m^2}\right) \tag{3.9}$$

Because the variance in each principal direction is given by the eigenvalues, $\sigma_m^2$ can be replaced by the corresponding eigenvalue $\lambda_m$.

**Quantization**

To be able to encode a training shape as an information theoretic message, all coordinates must first be quantized to a suitable accuracy $\Delta$. Following Eq. 3.9, the probability for a quantized value $\hat{b}_m = n\Delta, n \in \mathbb{Z}$ can be approximated by:

$$P(\hat{b}_m) \approx \frac{\Delta}{\sqrt{2\pi\lambda_m}} \exp\left(-\frac{\hat{b}_m^2}{2\lambda_m}\right) \tag{3.10}$$

As pointed out by Davies [52], this approximation has an error of less than one percent while $\lambda_m \geqslant 4\Delta^2$, hence a minimum $\lambda_{min}$ is defined for which the subsequent calculations remain faithful:

$$\lambda_{min} = 4\Delta^2 \tag{3.11}$$

The value for $\Delta$ should be chosen according to the expected noise on the training data.

**Description length**

The starting point for the formalization is Shannon's codeword length [208]: An information $a$ with the probability of occurrence $P(a)$ can be encoded in $\mathcal{L}$ bits using:

$$\mathcal{L} = -\log P(a) \tag{3.12}$$

Substituting $P(a)$ with $P(\hat{b}_m)$ from Eq. 3.10 results in the description length for one value $\hat{b}_m^{(i)}$:

$$\mathcal{L}(\hat{b}_m^{(i)}) = -\log \Delta + \log \sqrt{2\pi\lambda_m} + \frac{(\hat{b}_m^{(i)})^2}{2\lambda_m} \tag{3.13}$$

The description length for all values in one principal direction $m$ is the sum over all training samples:

$$\mathcal{L}_m = -n_s \log \Delta + n_s \log \sqrt{2\pi\lambda_m} + \sum_{i=1}^{n_s} \frac{(\hat{b}_m^{(i)})^2}{2\lambda_m}$$

$$= -n_s \log \Delta + \frac{n_s}{2} \log(2\pi\lambda_m) + \frac{1}{2\lambda_m} \sum_{i=1}^{n_s} (\hat{b}_m^{(i)})^2 \qquad (3.14)$$

In the limiting case $\Delta \to 0$, the quantized values approach the original values:

$$\hat{b}_m \to b_m \text{ and } \lambda_m \to \frac{1}{n_s} \sum_{i=1}^{n_s} (\hat{b}_m^{(i)})^2 \qquad (3.15)$$

Using this in (3.14) leads to:

$$\mathcal{L}_m^{(1)} = -n_s \log \Delta + \frac{n_s}{2} \log 2\pi + \frac{n_s}{2} \log \lambda_m + \frac{n_s}{2} \qquad (3.16)$$

A special case occurs if the eigenvalue $\lambda_m$ drops below the critical $\lambda_{min}$, as defined in (3.11). In this case, the probability for $\hat{b}_m$ is approximated using a distribution of $\lambda_{min}$. From (3.14) and (3.15) it follows:

$$\mathcal{L}_m^{(2)} = -n_s \log \Delta + \frac{n_s}{2} \log 2\pi + \frac{n_s}{2} \log \lambda_{min} + \frac{n_s}{2} \frac{\lambda_m}{\lambda_{min}} \qquad (3.17)$$

The entire dataset is transmitted by sending each principal direction separately, which leads to the final cost function of:

$$F = \sum_{m=1}^{n_s-1} \mathcal{L}_m \qquad (3.18)$$

In the original derivation [52], description length is composed of the length for data (similar to the formulation above) and the length of transmitting parameters. For each principal direction, the values of $\sigma_m$ are quantized with accuracy $\delta$, which for small $\lambda_m$ is given by $\sqrt{12\lambda_m/n_s}$. The description length for parameters is thus:

$$\mathcal{L}_{parameters} = \mathcal{L}_{\hat{\sigma}} + \mathcal{L}_\delta \qquad (3.19)$$

Since the description length of parameters plays only a minor role in the complete cost function, this part was omitted in the above derivation.

**Simplification**

To define an efficient cost function for optimization, the formulation from Eqs. 3.16 and 3.17 can be simplified by leaving out the constant terms which are equal for all models/correspondences. Further multiplication with $\frac{2}{n_s}$ yields:

$$\mathcal{L}_m = \begin{cases} \log \lambda_m + 1 & \text{for } \lambda_m \geqslant \lambda_{\min} \\ \log \lambda_{\min} + (\lambda_m/\lambda_{\min}) & \text{for } \lambda_m < \lambda_{\min} \end{cases} \qquad (3.20)$$

Subtracting $\log \lambda_{\min}$ then results in the same formulation that has been proposed by Thodberg [239]:

$$\mathcal{L}_m = \begin{cases} \log(\lambda_m/\lambda_{\min}) + 1 & \text{for } \lambda_m \geqslant \lambda_{\min} \\ \lambda_m/\lambda_{\min} & \text{for } \lambda_m < \lambda_{\min} \end{cases} \qquad (3.21)$$

Inserted in Eq. 3.18, this leads to the cost function utilized throughout this work.

### 3.3.2 Modifying correspondences

To optimize point correspondences with presented cost function, two possibilities are available: Changing the individual parameterizations $\Omega_i$ and maintaining a fixed set of global landmarks on the unit sphere, or modifying the individual landmark sets $\Psi_i$. In this work, the first alternative was chosen, which has the advantage that correspondences are valid for any set of points placed on the unit sphere. Therefore, it is possible to alter number and placement of landmarks on the unit sphere at any stage of the optimization, e.g. to better adapt the triangulation to the training shapes (more on this in Sec. 3.4).

To modify the individual parameterizations in an iterative optimization process, a transformation function of the type $\Omega' = \Phi(\Omega)$ is required. Davies et al. [55] use symmetric theta transformations for that purpose. Employing a wrapped Cauchy kernel with a certain width and amplitude, landmarks near the kernel position are spread over the sphere, while landmarks in other regions of the surface are compressed. By accumulating the effects of thousands of kernels at different positions, arbitrary parameterizations can be created.

While this re-parameterization method produces the required effect, it is an inefficient means of modifying surface parameterizations. The main disadvantage lies in global modification, i.e. adding one new kernel modifies all

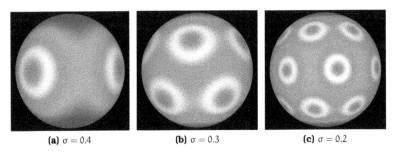

**(a)** $\sigma = 0.4$        **(b)** $\sigma = 0.3$        **(c)** $\sigma = 0.2$

**Figure 3.6:** Kernel configurations for $\sigma$ values of 0.4, 0.3 and 0.2. Red colors mark regions with large vertex movements, blue ones those with no modification.

landmark positions on the object. Intuitively, it would be desirable to keep established landmark correspondences stable. Therefore, a new method for modifying parameterization functions based on kernels with strictly local effects is presented below.

Assuming that a principal direction $(\Delta\theta, \Delta\phi)$ in which the vertices of a local neighborhood on the parameterization mesh should move to improve landmark correspondences is known, a Gaussian envelope function to change each spherical coordinate by $c(x, \sigma) \cdot (\Delta\theta, \Delta\phi)$ can be defined with

$$c(x, \sigma) = \begin{cases} e^{\frac{-x^2}{2\sigma^2}} - e^{\frac{-(3\sigma)^2}{2\sigma^2}} & \text{for } x < 3\sigma \\ 0 & \text{for } x \geqslant 3\sigma \end{cases} \tag{3.22}$$

Variable $x$ denotes the Euclidean distance between the center of the kernel and the specific vertex of the parameterization mesh, while $\sigma$ specifies the size of the kernel. The movements are cut off at $3\sigma$ to limit the range and keep the modification local. During the course of the optimization, $\sigma$ is decreased to optimize larger regions at the beginning and details at the end. Three examples for possible kernel configurations with different $\sigma$-values are shown in Fig. 3.6.

The proposed method of modification does not work if a kernel includes one of the poles of the spherical parameterization mesh ($\phi = 0$ or $\phi = \pi$) as vertices would all move either toward or away from this point, depending on $\Delta\phi$. Nevertheless, the positions of the different kernels have to change in the course of the optimization in order to guarantee an equal treatment for all vertices of the parameterization mesh. This limitation is overcome by

defining specific kernel configurations as shown in Fig. 3.6, which do not cover the pole sections of the sphere. By keeping these configurations fixed whilst rotating all parameterizations and the global landmark collection by a random rotation matrix, the relative kernel positions are changed without touching a pole. The random rotation matrices for these operations are acquired using the method described by Arvo [3].

### 3.3.3 The optimization scheme

Before presenting the details of optimization, let us briefly recapitulate how landmark positions influence the eigenvalues $\lambda_m$ of the SSM and thus the cost function. For every sample of the training set, landmark points are defined by a single vector $\mathbf{x}$, storing the coordinates for landmark $i$ at $(x_{3i}, x_{3i+1}, x_{3i+2})$. The vectors of all training samples form the columns of the landmark configuration matrix $\mathbf{L}$. In order to calculate the PCA, a singular value decomposition (SVD) is used instead of an eigenvector decomposition of the covariance matrix of $\mathbf{L}$ (as suggested by Cootes et al. [43]). According to Kalman [124], this method is numerically more stable and thus more accurate when the covariance matrix is ill-conditioned. The singular value decomposition is defined as follows:

**Definition 2** *Any* $m \times n$ *real matrix* $\mathbf{A}$ *with* $m \geqslant n$ *can be written as the product*

$$\mathbf{A} = \mathbf{U}\mathbf{D}\mathbf{V}^{\mathbf{T}} \qquad\qquad (3.23)$$

*where* $\mathbf{U}$ *and* $\mathbf{V}$ *are column orthogonal matrices of size* $m \times n$ *and* $n \times n$, *respectively, and* $\mathbf{D}$ *is a* $n \times n$ *diagonal matrix. Then* $\mathbf{U}$ *holds the eigenvectors of the matrix* $\mathbf{A}\mathbf{A}^{\mathbf{T}}$ *and* $\mathbf{D}^{\mathbf{2}}$ *the corresponding eigenvalues.*

Without calculating the covariance matrix, the PCA can thus be obtained by the SVD of the matrix:

$$\mathbf{A} = \frac{1}{\sqrt{n_s - 1}}(\mathbf{L} - \bar{\mathbf{L}}), \qquad\qquad (3.24)$$

where $n_s$ is the number of samples and $\bar{\mathbf{L}}$ a matrix with all columns set to $\bar{\mathbf{x}}$. In addition to increased accuracy, the matrices $\mathbf{U}$ and $\mathbf{V}$ allow calculating gradient information for the eigenvalues, as explained in the next paragraph.

**Derivation of gradients**

Given a kernel at a certain position, the direction $(\Delta\theta, \Delta\phi)$ for the movement that minimizes the cost function is needed. Since all modifications of the parameterization change landmark positions on the training sample, the first step is to quantify the effect landmark movements have on the cost function. As shown in [72], the work of Papadopoulo and Lourakis on estimating the Jacobian of the SVD [182] can be used for that purpose.

Given the centered and un-biased landmark configuration matrix $\mathbf{A}$ from Eq. 3.24, the derivative for the m-th singular value $d_m$ is calculated by:

$$\frac{\partial d_m}{\partial a_{ij}} = u_{im} \cdot v_{jm} \tag{3.25}$$

The scalars $u_{im}$ and $v_{jm}$ are elements of the matrices $\mathbf{U}$ and $\mathbf{V}$ from (3.23). Since the employed cost function uses $\lambda_m = d_m^2$, gradients can be derived as:

$$\frac{\partial F}{\partial a_{ij}} = \sum_m \frac{\partial \mathcal{L}_m}{\partial a_{ij}} \quad \text{with} \quad \frac{\partial \mathcal{L}_m}{\partial a_{ij}} = \begin{cases} 2u_{im}v_{jm}/d_m & \text{for } \lambda_m \geqslant \lambda_{min} \\ 2d_m u_{im}v_{jm}/\lambda_{min} & \text{for } \lambda_m < \lambda_{min} \end{cases} \tag{3.26}$$

This derivation yields a 3D gradient for every landmark, revealing the influence of its movements on the cost function. Two examples of the resulting gradient fields are visualized in Fig. 3.7.

**Putting it all together**

The final step requires the transformation of the calculated gradient fields into optimal kernel movements $\mathbf{k} = (\Delta\theta, \Delta\phi)$ on the parameterization mesh. Using the chain rule results in:

$$\frac{\partial F}{\partial \mathbf{k}} = \frac{\partial F}{\partial a_{ij}} \frac{\partial a_{ij}}{\partial \mathbf{k}} \tag{3.27}$$

Finite differences are employed to estimate the surface gradients $\partial a_{ij}/\partial\mathbf{k}$.

Both Davies [52] and Thodberg [239] describe cases in which the optimization can lead to landmarks piling up in certain regions or collapsing to a point. Davies keeps one shape as a master example with fixed landmarks to prevent this effect while Thodberg suggests adding a stabilizing term to the cost function. The problematic behavior was not observed with the presented new re-parameterization, despite the lack of employing these methods.

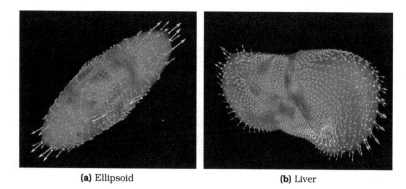

(a) Ellipsoid                    (b) Liver

**Figure 3.7:** Gradients of the MDL cost function visualized for two sample shapes. The value of the directional derivative is color-coded ranging from blue for weak gradients to red for the strongest gradients.

In addition to modifying the mapping functions $\Omega_i$ by re-parameterization, other variables which influence landmark positions can be included in the optimization. The rotation of each mapping $\Omega_i$ determines the position of the first landmark on the training shape and the relative orientation of all others. Calculating gradients for rotating the parameterization mesh around the three Euclidean axes and using those instead of the surface gradients $\partial a_{ij}/\partial \mathbf{k}$ in (3.27) constitutes an efficient method to optimize this variable.

Other possibilities for optimization include scale and rotation of the individual training shapes, which are usually determined by a generalized procrustes matching. While scale is optimized in the presented procedure, no significant improvements in the resulting cost function values were observed due to this step. Figure 3.8 shows some pseudocode for the final optimization scheme.

## 3.4 Landmark redistribution

As described in Sec. 3.2, initial parameterization functions are angle-preserving to provide optimal conditions for the presented optimization scheme. However, since these inital versions are changed constantly during the optimization by warping with varying kernels, the final outcome of a parameteriza-

---

**Algorithm 3.3.1:** OPTIMIZECORRESPONDENCES()

**procedure** OPTIMIZELOCALKERNELS(LoD)
  **for** $i \leftarrow 0$ **to** numSamples
    **do for** $k \leftarrow 0$ **to** numKernels$_{LoD}$
    **do** warpGradient$_{i,k} \leftarrow$ GETKERNELDERIVATIVE(LoD, i, k)
  **for** $i \leftarrow 0$ **to** numSamples
    **do for** $k \leftarrow 0$ **to** numKernels$_{LoD}$
    **do** params$_i \leftarrow$ WARP(params$_i$, LoD, k,
                 warpStep $\cdot$ warpGradient$_{i,k}$)


**procedure** OPTIMIZESTARTVALUES()
  **for** $i \leftarrow 0$ **to** numSamples
    **do** rotGradient$_i \leftarrow$ GETROTATIONALDERIVATIVE(i)
  **for** $i \leftarrow 0$ **to** numSamples
    **do** params$_i \leftarrow$ ROTATE(params$_i$, rotStep $\cdot$ rotGradient$_i$)


costs $\leftarrow$ EVALUATECOSTFUNCTION()
iteration $\leftarrow 0$
LoD $\leftarrow 0$
**repeat**
  OPTIMIZELOCALKERNELS(LoD)
  BUILDMODEL()
  OPTIMIZESTARTVALUES()
  ROTATEPARAMETERIZATIONSANDLANDMARKS()
  BUILDMODEL()
  iteration $\leftarrow$ iteration $+ 1$
  **if** $(iteration modulo 50) = 0$
          $\begin{cases} c \leftarrow \text{EVALUATECOSTFUNCTION}() \\ \textbf{if } (costs - c) < \epsilon \\ \quad \textbf{then } LoD \leftarrow LoD + 1 \\ costs \leftarrow c \end{cases}$
  **then**
**until** $(LoD = maxLoD)$

---

**Figure 3.8:** Pseudocode to optimize landmark correspondences for the construction of a SSM.

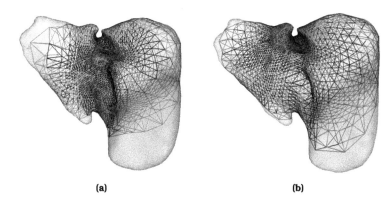

**(a)**                                                     **(b)**

**Figure 3.9:** Landmarks and corresponding triangulations on a training shape for the liver model (displayed transparently). For the shape in (a), correspondence optimization was started with conformal parameterizations, for (b) with diffusion mapping. Both versions exhibit considerable variation in landmark density, leading to deficient shape representations. The two-dimensional display may evoke the impression of vertices postitioned inside the volume, but all landmarks are located on the surface of the training shape.

tion is unpredictable and will generally not feature any specific properties. For shape model construction, the resulting area deformation of the final parameterization is of special interest, as it directly influences the distribution of landmarks on the training shapes and thus on the SSM. Although landmarks are distributed equally over the surface of the spherical parameterization mesh, density of the mapped positions on training shapes will usually vary widely.

This issue becomes critical when landmarks are spread so sparsely in certain regions that triangulation does not represent the shape accurately (Fig. 3.9). A solution to this problem is to change the global landmark set $\Psi$: Since point correspondences are specified by the individual parameterizations, reconfiguring landmarks on the sphere will maintain these correspondences whilst simulaneously generating new triangulations for all training shapes. In this section, methods are presented which reconfigure landmarks after or during the optimization process in order to achieve an equal distribution of landmarks on the final model.

### 3.4.1 Remeshing surfaces

The problem of finding new landmark positions for a shape model is closely related to the problem of remeshing a polygonal surface, i.e. finding new vertex positions and a new triangulation for a single shape. Since this is an active field of research in computer graphics, there exists a multitude of different approaches for remeshing (e.g. Peyre and Cohen [190], Surazhsky and Gotsman [232], and Vorsatz et al. [256]). In order to utilize one of these methods for reconfiguring the landmarks of the shape model, a way to incorporate the shape variation into the process is required. In this thesis, this was accomplished by using the entire collection of training meshes as input (from which all the variance information is derived). The basis for the procedure is the work by Alliez et al. [1], which is briefly resumed below.

First, the input mesh is converted into a collection of two-dimensional maps in parameter space. These maps define the desired vertex densities for the entire surface and can be set up to any desired distribution, e.g. most economic representation (i.e. a sparser net of vertices in regions with lower curvature) or a uniform vertex distribution. The higher the values in a certain area of the map, the denser the vertices will be placed in the corresponding surface area of the mesh. In order to reach an equal distribution of vertices, a distortion ratio is computed for each triangle of the mesh, defined as the area of the triangle on the input mesh divided by the area on the 2D map. The triangle is then drawn on the map with the value of this ratio as color, leading to a map of the area distortion on the shape (Fig. 3.10(a)). Subsequently, this map is dithered with a predefined number of points using an error diffusion algorithm as the one presented by Ostromoukhov [181]. Positions of all points are mapped back to the mesh and give a first solution for an equal distribution of vertices. The new vertex connections are determined by a Delaunay triangulation on the 2D maps (Fig. 3.10(b)).

In the case of multiple maps, the vertices of all parts must be reconnected for the new mesh. This is accomplished by a separate, one-dimensional dithering process along the boundary of all maps. Each resulting pixel is inserted in both maps adjacent to the respective boundary. These constrained vertices are connected to the existing points inside the map forming a convex triangulation (the outer circle in Fig. 3.10(b)). When mapping back the vertices to the mesh, corresponding boundary points result in the identical location and are stitched together. In a final relaxation step, all vertices are pulled along the surface toward their direct neighbors, using a

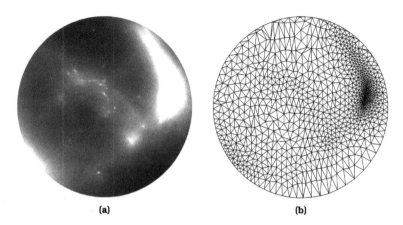

          **(a)**                                **(b)**

**Figure 3.10:** Area distortion and resulting landmark positions for one half-sphere. The ratio between area on model surface and area in parameter space in stored as a 2D map (a). After dithering the map, the resulting white pixels are connected by a 2D Delaunay triangulation (b). When this geometry is mapped back to the sphere and joined with the other half-sphere, it forms the prototype for the new landmark configuration.

force proportional to the respective length of the edge connecting the points. This smoothes any random perturbations that could have arisen during the dithering or the stitching process.

### 3.4.2 Adaptation to SSMs

The adaptation of this remeshing approach to statistical shape models works as follows: instead of a single mesh that has to be remeshed, an entire collection of training shapes has to be triangulated with the same topology. Parameterizations for these meshes exist, albeit of spherical topology. To obtain the required two-dimensional images, each parameterization is separated in two half-spheres and stereographic projection is used to create two disk-like patches for each mesh (Fig. 3.11). Since the spherical parameterizations correspond over all shapes, the two-dimensional maps also match. Thus, all patches representing the same side of the sphere can be averaged, yielding two control maps on which the dithering is performed. The resulting landmark densities are optimal to represent the entire collec-

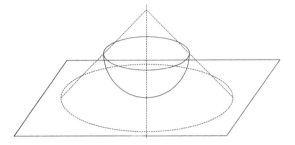

**Figure 3.11:** Stereographic projection from half-sphere to plane. All lines of projection starts at the highest point of the full sphere.

tion of training shapes, which means that they also represent the shape model in an optimal way. An example of a successfully reconfigured training shape is displayed in Fig. 3.12.

### 3.4.3 The modified optimization scheme

In Chapter 6, several experiments to determine the best method to incorporate the presented remeshing algorithm in the gradient-based optimization framework are described. In particular, there is the choice between applying the landmark redistribution once, after the standard optimization described in Sec. 3.3 has converged, and applying it continuously during the optimization. In the latter case, landmarks are reorganized every 10 iterations, which has the advantage that the cost function is always evaluated on a model with equally distributed landmarks. Both methods are expected to produce better models than those obtained by the standard optimization approach (without reconfiguration).

## 3.5 Performance measures

In order to estimate the quality of the presented model construction scheme and the impact of landmark reconfiguration, an objective performance index for evaluation is needed. Davies [52] describes the measures of compactness, generalization ability and specificity to compare the performance of different models.

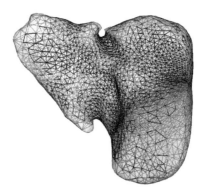

**Figure 3.12:** The same shape as in Fig. 3.9 with a reconfigured landmark set. All landmarks are equally spread over the surface, leading to an accurate representation of the shape data.

Compactness is the sum of eigenvalues for the statistical model and is displayed as a function of the number of modes that are added (beginning with the largest one). While this is interesting to assess the amount of variance in a shape model, it does not seem to be a fair measure to compare different SSMs. The MDL approach for correspondence assumes that lower eigenvalues result in better models and explicitly minimizes them, which gives it a large advantage for this measure. For this reason, focus is laid on the less biased remaining two measures throughout this thesis.

Generalization ability quantifies the capability of the model to represent new shapes. It can be estimated by performing a series of leave-one-out tests on the training set, measuring the difference of the omitted training shape to the closest match of the reduced model. Specificity describes the validity of the shapes the model produces. The value is estimated by generating random parameter values from a normal distribution with zero mean and the respective standard deviation from the PCA. The difference of the generated shape to the closest match of the training set is averaged over a large number of runs. Both measures are defined as functions of the number of modes or parameters used by the model and displayed as piecewise linear graphs. Smaller values indicate better models.

To quantify the difference between two shapes $\mathbf{x}$ and $\mathbf{y}$ with landmark i located at the position $\mathbf{l}_x(i)$ respective $\mathbf{l}_y(i)$, originally the sum of squares error was used [52]:

$$d_{sse}(\mathbf{x}, \mathbf{y}) = \sum_{i=1}^{n} |\mathbf{l}_x(i) - \mathbf{l}_y(i)|^2 \qquad (3.28)$$

In subsequent studies [228], this metric was replaced by the mean absolute distance, stabilizing it in regard to changes of the number of landmarks n:

$$d_{mad}(\mathbf{x}, \mathbf{y}) = \frac{1}{n} \sum_{i=1}^{n} |\mathbf{l}_x(i) - \mathbf{l}_y(i)| \qquad (3.29)$$

### 3.5.1 Pitfalls of model evaluation

When using these measures to compare the performance of different shape models, one has to assure that evaluation is valid and unbiased. In the following, some of the common pitfalls are listed, which are prone to causing invalid results and deserve special attention.

### Scale

Since current evaluation measures are based on distances between landmarks, the models to be compared must have exactly the same size. But how can we define a standard size for the evaluation if all training samples are scaled with individual factors before building the landmark matrix $\mathbf{L}$? To maintain model size at a stable level, one possibility is to scale the mean shape to feature a RMS radius of $r = 1/\sqrt{n}$ [239]. In this case, changing the number of landmarks n obviously leads to a different model size, but varying only landmark positions does as well (since both the shape center and the average distance to it will change, leading to a different RMS radius). An example of that problem is shown in Fig. 3.13. A more accurate method is to leave training samples at their original sizes and let the model scale for a best fit. However, this procedure is not suited for inputs of different sizes as all errors will be weighted with the input scale. For the evaluation in this thesis, all models are scaled to a common size determined by the input meshes. Since variations of the individual scale factors $s_i$ should be possible during optimization, their average is constrained to a stable level: $\sum_{i=1}^{n} s_i/n = 1$.

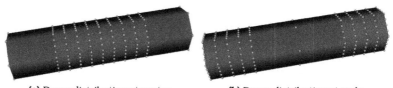

**(a)** Dense distribution at center          **(b)** Dense distribution at ends

**Figure 3.13:** Two identical shape models with different landmark distributions. When scaling both models to a fixed RMS radius, model (b) will end up much smaller than model (a). The reason is that its landmarks are concentrated more at the ends, thus the RMS radius (measured from all landmarks) appears larger, which leads to more down-sizing.

### Number of landmarks

When measuring distance between shapes with the sum of squares error, it is obvious that both models must have the same number of landmarks. Using mean absolute distance instead seems to remedy this problem. However, models with a larger number of landmarks naturally capture more detail and thus more variance of the shape. Thus, they face a disadvantage when it comes to a comparison with a coarser model. To conclude, only models with the same number of landmarks should be compared using the current evaluation methods.

### Landmark distribution

The most unexpected problem is the one of different landmark distributions. Any two non-identical models will have their landmarks located at different positions. In addition to the consequences on scaling described above, the variance of a shape model varies considerably over the surface (Fig. 3.14). If two shape models with similar mean shapes and displacement vectors are compared, the model with a larger part of landmarks in low-variance areas will always produce better performance values. One approach to solve this, is to adjust the distribution of one model to match that of the second one. While this method does work, it implicates a slight disadvantage for the model with the changed distribution, since its landmarks were not optimized for these specific locations.

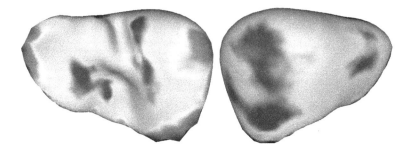

**Figure 3.14:** Color-coded standard deviation for all landmarks on the surface of the liver model. The values range from 1.3 (dark blue) to 5.2 (bright red). The inhomogeneous concentration of high-variance areas at protruding bulges is clearly visible.

### 3.5.2 A new metric

The depicted problems of evaluating shape models originate in the way the difference between two model instances is measured. Both sum of squares error as well as mean absolute distance are metrics focused on landmarks and landmark distance. However, when using shape models in image analysis, the main interest often lies in the resulting segmentation (i.e. the volume encompassed by the model), not in the exact landmark locations. In reference to performance evaluation in image segmentation [176], there are several metrics that seem to be better suited for the task of shape comparison, e.g.:

- Hausdorff distance: this metric measures the maximum distance between two surfaces. If $d(x, y)$ is the distance between two points, the Hausdorff distance between two surfaces $X$ and $Y$ is defined as:

$$D_{HD}(X, Y) = \max(h(X, Y), h(Y, X)) \quad \text{with} \quad h(X, Y) = \max_{x \in X} \min_{y \in Y} d(x, y)$$

(3.30)

- Average squared surface distance: since the Hausdorff distance is very sensitive to outliers, an alternative is to average the squared distances over both surfaces:

$$D_{ASD}(X, Y) = \frac{1}{2} \left( \sum_{x \in X} \min_{y \in Y} d^2(x, y) + \sum_{y \in Y} \min_{x \in X} d^2(y, x) \right)$$

(3.31)

- Volumetric overlap: there are several measures to quantify the similarity between two volumes A and B, a popular one being the Tanimoto coefficient[236] (also known as Jaccard coefficient):

$$C_T = \frac{|A \cap B|}{|A \cup B|} \tag{3.32}$$

  The Tanimoto coefficient yields 1 if both shapes are identical and 0 for no overlap at all. To transform the measure into a distance metric, the obvious way is to negate it as in $D_T = 1 - C_T$.

From a computational point of view, measuring surface distances is more complex and time-consuming than measuring overlap, even considering that the surface of the model has to be converted into a binary volume first. Especially for the evaluation of specificity (which involves 100,000s of shape comparisons), computational requirements have to be taken into account. For this reason, the Tanimoto coefficient was chosen as a volumetric overlap measure. For the computation of generalization ability and specificity, the generated instances of the model are compared to the original input training shapes, not their model approximations. This procedure ensures that the metric measures unbiased performance and is sensitive to deficient shape representation as shown in Fig. 3.9.

# 4 Local Appearance Models

> *Mathematics is looking for patterns.*
> — *Richard P. Feynman, "What is science?" (1966)*

Modeling the shape of an object of interest is merely one part of a knowledge-based segmentation approach – the other being modeling of the gray-value appearance of the object in order to robustly recognize it in unseen images. In the first section of this chapter (Sec. 4.1), several methods on how to model this appearance at the boundary of the object of interest are described. This is followed by a description of the clustering method that is used to increase the number of training samples for each model in Sec. 4.2. Finally, a procedure for estimating the performance of different appearance models without utilizing them for segmentation is introduced in Sec. 4.3.

## 4.1 Basic appearance models

In this section, the different appearance models used in this thesis are presented. All models are local, i.e. they represent the appearance around a single landmark point of the SSM. In order to employ an appearance model for segmentation, it must be able to compare a position in a new image with the learned appearance and output the corresponding fitting costs $c_f$. The more similar the tested position is to the learned appearance, the lower these costs are (zero costs indicates a perfect fit). For the basic models discussed here, there is no defined upper limit for costs. In addition to the fitting costs, it is generally convenient if the appearance model can also output an estimate for the probability $p_b$ of a boundary at the tested location. Obviously, the output for this probability has to be limited to $[0, 1]$ and higher costs have to lead to lower probabilities.

### 4.1.1 Gaussian intensity profile model

The plain intensity profile was one of the first statistical appearance models used for segmentation [34, 35]. At the modeled landmark, an intensity

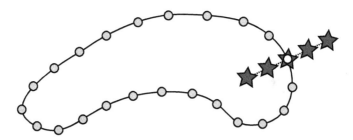

**Figure 4.1:** 2D example of an intensity profile to model appearance. The SSM is represented by a number of landmarks, each with its own appearance model. Assuming a profile of length 5 for the white landmark, intensity values are sampled from the image at the locations of the blue stars.

profile g is sampled perpendicular to the boundary. Generally, one value is sampled at the boundary itself and $m$ values are sampled at different positions towards the inside and the outside of the object, leading to a profile size of $2m+1$ samples. Common numbers for $m$ vary between 1 and 5, leading to profile lengths between 3 and 11 samples. There is a fixed distance $\Delta$ between two consecutive samples, which should always be measured in physical coordinates (i.e. mm, not voxels) in order to be able to apply the model to images of different resolutions. Figure 4.1 shows a simple 2D example of an intensity profile model.

During training of the appearance model, one profile is sampled at each landmark in each training image. For each landmark, all resulting profiles are combined into one model. The general assumption is that appearance can be modeled by a Gaussian distribution. Thus, the mean profile $\bar{g}$ and the standard covariance matrix $\Sigma$ are computed for each landmark. The similarity of a test profile g with the modeled distribution can be determined by calculating the corresponding Mahalanobis distance $d_M$, given by:

$$d_M(g) = (g - \bar{g})\Sigma^{-1}(g - \bar{g}) \qquad (4.1)$$

Conveniently, the probability of g belonging to the modeled distribution (and thus to the boundary of the SSM) can directly be estimated from the Mahalanobis distance:

$$p_b(g) = \alpha e^{-0.5 d_M(g)} \qquad (4.2)$$

where $\alpha \in [0, 1]$ is a scaling factor that determines the probability of the mean profile belonging to the distribution. As this value is dependent on

the gray-value appearance of the background (which is not considered in the standard approach), it can only be estimated by experiment. The fitting costs $c_f(g)$ are directly derived from the probabilities by:

$$c_f(g) = 1 - p_b(g) \qquad (4.3)$$

A modification of the plain intensity profile is the normalized intensity profile $g_n$, which scales all profile samples so that their absolute values sum up to one:

$$g_n(i) = \frac{g(i)}{\sum_{j=-m}^{m} |g(j)|} \qquad (4.4)$$

where $g(i)$ and $g_n(i)$ indicate the i-th sample in the respective profile.

### 4.1.2 Gaussian gradient profile model

Together with the intensity profile, the gradient profile was also introduced as one of the first appearance models [34, 35]. As the name suggests, a gradient profile stores the differences between neighboring intensity values, i.e. $g'(i) = g(i + 1) - g(i - 1)$. To deliver a gradient profile of size $2m + 1$, $2m + 3$ values have to be sampled from the image in order to estimate the gradient at the end points. Fitting costs are calculated as for the intensity profile model, using the Mahalanobis distance (Eq. 4.1). Obviously, it is also possible to normalize gradient profiles as described by Eq. 4.4.

### 4.1.3 Non-linear intensity profile model

The two approaches described above for appearance modeling have two weak points: first, it is assumed that all profiles follow a Gaussian distribution (which is not always the case with real images), and second, no information about competing models representing non-boundary areas are taken into account. Both shortcomings are remedied by the non-linear classifier approach that has been presented for the analysis of 2D images by de Bruijne et al. [60].

In this approach, a k-nearest-neighbor (kNN) classifier is used to distinguish between boundary and non-boundary samples. During training, a number of additional profiles have to be sampled at locations other than the true landmark positions in order to model the non-boundary class. This is accomplished by shifting the sample location perpendicular to the object boundary, m steps towards the inside and m steps towards the outside of

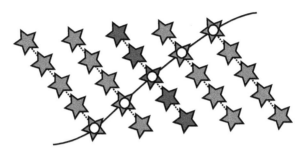

**Figure 4.2:** Visualization of the training process for a non-linear profile model. At each landmark a number of shifted profiles are sampled, marked as *boundary* (blue) or *non-boundary* (red). For displaying purposes the shifted profiles are shown at different landmark positions.

the object. Each step should have the same size as the profile spacing $\Delta$. An example for the training process is shown in Fig. 4.2. Storing all training profiles together with their class, the fitting costs of a test profile can be determined by searching the k nearest neighbors (using the Euclidean metric here) and evaluating the ratio of boundary profiles $b_k(g)$ among them. A high amount of boundary profiles should result in low fitting costs $c_f$, leading to:

$$c_f(g) = 1 - \frac{b_k(g)}{k} \tag{4.5}$$

The obvious way to estimate the boundary probability would be to use $p_b(g) = \frac{b_k(g)}{k}$. However, zero probabilities should be avoided for further processing. Therefore, a moderated kNN-classifer [131] was chosen, which defines:

$$p_b(g) = \frac{b_k(g) + 1}{k + 2} \tag{4.6}$$

As for the previously presented appearance models, all sample profiles can also be normalized prior to using them.

### 4.1.4 Non-linear gradient profile model

A variant of the non-linear intensity profile model is the corresponding gradient profile model. As for the Gaussian gradient profile, two additional values must be sampled at the ends of the profile to estimate the gradients

located there. This version also works with the original gradients and with all gradients normalized to 1 over the profile.

### 4.1.5 Histogram region model

While profile models can describe the boundary appearance very efficiently, the amount of data reduction may actually be too much for certain data. If images are too noisy, small changes of sample location or orientation may change the values of the sampled profile substantially. In order to obtain a more robust boundary description, it is necessary to incorporate more information from the landmark appearance into the model.

An alternative approach to profile sampling is to collect data from an entire local image volume, e.g. from a cylinder spanned around the landmark normal. To analyze the collected data, histogram statistics are employed, which have been shown an effective way of modeling object appearance in several recent publications [84, 24]. First, the sampled volume is divided into two regions (inside and outside of the object), and histograms are created for each one individually. Subsequently, both histograms are concatenated, forming what is called a *dual histogram* (Fig. 4.3). During training, dual histograms are sampled from all training images and stored on a per-landmark basis. To determine fitting costs for a test position x in a new image, the dual histogram $h_x$ is sampled and compared to all corresponding stored histograms $h_i$. The employed comparison metric is the $L_1$ distance, which has been shown to be well suitable for histogram matching [25]. The minimum of all comparisons represents the final costs:

$$c_f(x) = \min_i |h_i - h_x| \qquad (4.7)$$

In order to efficiently collect intensity data for the histogram, a set of mask images is generated. The first mask consists of a vertically oriented cylinder of a specified diameter, where a value of 1 labels the upper half and a value of 2 labels the lower half. This template mask is rotated to align the cylinder to a number of equally sampled directions, generating the other mask images. Directions are obtained by forming the vectors from the center of an icosahedron to all its vertices (or all vertices of a sub-divided icosahedron, depending on the desired angular resolution). To collect histogram data around a specific landmark, the mask that best approximates the corresponding normal vector is shifted to the respective location in the image. Subsequently, image voxels can be assigned to inner and outer histogram according to the corresponding labels in the mask.

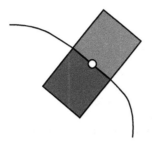 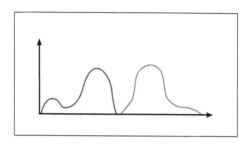

**Figure 4.3:** Dual histogram appearance model. A certain region around a landmark is divided into inner (blue) and outer (red) part. Intensity histograms are sampled from both regions and concatenated to a single function.

## 4.2 Clustering

As all statistical models, the models describing the local gray-value appearance around a landmark will usually improve when given more training data. If the number of input images is fixed, one possibility to increase the amount of training data is to combine information from different landmarks to build one clustered model. Since neighboring landmarks often exhibit very similar appearance, the model does not lose its specificity when joining the respective data. It is even possible that the appearance of landmarks on two opposing sides of the object of interest is very similar, e.g. when the same tissue types are present at both locations. For this reason, clustering does not rely on positional information, but exclusively on the feature vectors (e.g. intensity profiles) describing the appearance.

The original input to the clustering process is a large number of feature vectors $f_{ij}$, where index $i$ indicates the training image and $j$ the landmark. The output should consist of several sets of landmarks to build one clustered appearance model for each set. For the clustering process, this implicates that all feature vectors from the same landmark $j$ must be assigned to the same cluster. In this work, the problem is solved by calculating average feature vectors $f_j$ for each landmark (over all training images $i$) and use these in the clustering process.

The method used for the actual clustering is the mean shift technique described by Comaniciu and Meer [29]. Here, a number of different points in feature space (either chosen randomly or by taking the position of given samples) are chosen as starting points for the process. For each of these

points, a new position is calculated by averaging all samples within a defined radius around them (the kernel region). By iterating this procedure, all mean positions are shifted along trajectories pointing towards local maxima of the sample density. Any sample passed by a trajectory is assigned to the peak where the specific trajectory ends, thus joining to several clusters. Figure 4.4 shows a 2D example of the method.

The mean shift algorithm can be adapted to a given problem by varying the radius of the kernel used for averaging the feature vectors. The larger this radius, the smoother the density estimate will be, resulting in less clusters. Moreover, a minimum cluster size can be specified, and all clusters that do not reach this number will be assigned to the closest larger cluster. By changing these two parameters, almost arbitrary numbers of clusters can be produced for a given data set.

## 4.3 Performance measures

Having the choice between different appearance models with varying parameters, being able to estimate their performance for a given image analysis problem is of great practical importance. The standard approach for this evaluation is to run a search algorithm with the respective appearance model and assess the outcome of the segmentation. By this procedure, the performance of a certain type of model can be estimated accurately. However, it is not possible to deduce the performance of the individual models independently for each landmark. The latter information would open up possibilities like weighting individual appearance models during the search according to their performance, or even combine different appearance model for one shape model by selecting the best option for each landmark.

### 4.3.1 Benchmarking by simulated search

The solution proposed in this work for the indivdual performance assessment is to simulate the SSM search on images where the true segmentation is known and to analyze the cost function responses of the different appearance models during the process. This method can be applied in cross-validation style, omitting a number of training images from the construction of the appearance models and using these as test set for validation.

Benchmarking functions as follows: in all images of the test set, fitting costs $c_f$ of the analyzed appearance model are calculated at the true boundary position and at 2K positions shifted towards the inside and outside of the object of interest (along the respective normal vector). To simulate realistic search conditions, the true boundary position is randomized around each landmark j with a uniform distribution in the polygon determined by the direct neighbors of j. In addition, the employed normal vectors are randomized with a standard deviation of $\sigma = 10$ degrees. This way, a number of R tests is run for each landmark in every image of the test set (R = 30 is employed throughout this work).

Regarding cost function response $c_f$ as a function of the displacement $k \in [-K..K]$, good appearance models should deliver a minimum value $c_f$ at $k = 0$ and high costs for all $k \neq 0$. Starting from this premise, the performance $\xi_r$ of one test r is evaluated by a weighted sum of differences between the fitting costs at the true position $c_f(0)$ and the ones at shifted positions $c_f(k)$:

$$\xi_r = \left( \sum_{k=-K}^{K} |k|^d \left( c_f(k) - c_f(0) \right) \right) / \left( \sum_{k=-K}^{K} |k|^d \right) \tag{4.8}$$

where d determines the influence of the shifting distance – d = 1 is used for all experiments in this thesis. As true position and normal vector are perturbed randomly, each test r will result in a slightly different $\xi_r$. By averaging the results over all tests, a performance index $\xi$ is estimated for each landmark. The larger $\xi$, the better the appearance model can differentiate between boundary and background. Random fitting costs result in $\xi = 0$, and a negative $\xi$ (which should rarely occur) implies that the appearance model systematically misplaces the true boundary. To be able to compare models of different types with each other, it is desirable to normalize the performance index to $\xi \in [-1..1]$. This can be accomplished by normalizing the individual cost functions $c_f$ to $[0..1]$.

### 4.3.2 Normalizing cost function response

To normalize the cost function $c_f$ of a given appearance model to lie in the interval $[0..1]$, minimum $c_{fmin}$ and maximum fitting costs $c_{fmax}$ the model typically delivers have to be known. The normalized fitting costs $c'_f$ can then

be calculated by:

$$c_f' = \begin{cases} 0 & \text{for } c_f \leqslant c_{fmin} \\ 1 & \text{for } c_f \geqslant c_{fmax} \\ \frac{c_f - c_{fmin}}{c_{fmax} - c_{fmin}} & \text{else} \end{cases} \tag{4.9}$$

The minimum and maximum values used here are estimated during a run of the simulated search detailed above. In the process of evaluating cost function response at many different locations, all $c_f$ for one landmark appearance model are collected in an ordered set. $c_{fmin}$ is then set to the 1%-quantile of this collection and $c_{fmax}$ to the 99% quantile. Using the thus normalized fitting costs $c_f'$ in Eq. 4.8 yields the normalized performance index utilized for all experiments in this thesis.

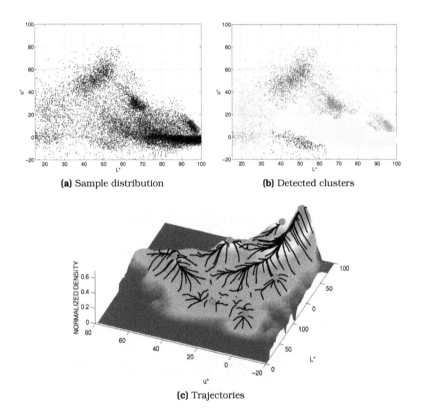

**(a)** Sample distribution          **(b)** Detected clusters

**(c)** Trajectories

**Figure 4.4:** Example for mean shift clustering in 2D feature space (all images from Comaniciu and Meer [29]). The data set in (a) is decomposed into the clusters shown in (b). The trajectories of the underlying mean shift procedure climb to the local maxima of the density estimate (c) – all samples encountered on these paths will be assigned to the end-points (marked with red dots).

# 5 Image Analysis Using Statistical Models

> *With four parameters I can fit an elephant,*
> *and with five I can make him wiggle his trunk.*
>
> — *John von Neumann*

This chapter presents a segmentation procedure for volumetric images which is based on statistical models of shape and appearance described in previous chapters. As outlined in Sec. 2.6, a typical approach for this problem is to adjust pose and shape parameters of the geometric model until the combined fitting costs of the appearance models are minimized. Since the resulting cost function generally features many local minima, an initial positioning close to the true location is essential for the correct convergence of local optimization schemes.

To accomplish the required initialization, one possibility is employing a manual approach as described in Sec. 5.1. As an alternative, an automatic method for the task which is based on global optimization is presented in Sec. 5.2. Using one of these approaches for a rough initialization, a local search algorithm built on techniques from deformable surface models is employed to extract the final contours of the object of interest – this method is described in Sec. 5.3. Section 5.4 presents a weighting scheme for appearance models which can be used in a variant of the local search, potentially improving segmentation results. The chapter concludes with a description of performance measures that can be used to evaluate the quality of obtained segmentations.

## 5.1 Manual initialization

To initialize the local search algorithm manually, it is sufficient to supply a suitable similarity transform which maps the model close to the object of interest. This transform can be specified interactively using the following procedure. After loading a new dataset and chosing the desired type of segmentation (e.g. liver from CT or heart from MRI), the corresponding mean

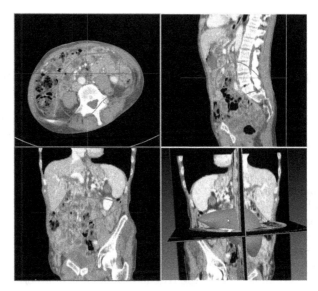

**Figure 5.1:** Graphical user interface to specify the inital similarity transform of the SSM. The user can translate the shape model by dragging the mouse with the left button, rotate it by using the right button and scale it by using the center button.

model is displayed in the center of the image. The user can then work with the mouse to align the centers of model and object of interest and to adjust rotation and scale of the model. All interaction can take place in any of the three image planes and in the 3D view (Fig. 5.1). The entire process takes typically less than ten seconds and is finished by pressing a button that starts the local search.

## 5.2 Automatic initialization

Although manual initialization is the most reliable method for setting the initial transform, there are applications where automatic approaches are in advantage, e.g. when a large number of images should be analyzed in a row. One possibility to initialize the SSM without user interaction is to perform a global search of the shape model in this image. For this task, an algo-

---

**Algorithm 5.2.1:** OPTIMIZE()

INITIALIZEPOPULATION()
**repeat**
  EVALUATEFITNESS()
  SELCETIONBYRANDOMSAMPLING()
  GAUSSIANMUTATION()
**until** (end)

---

**Figure 5.2:** Pseudocode for the used evolutionary algorithm.

rithm based on the concepts of evolutionary programming [81] and evolution strategies [205] is used in this work. Although these two methods were developed independently from each other, they differ only in details and share most of the important properties. Both are global search algorithms maintaining a population of different solutions which evolve by following the "survival of the fittest" rule: a higher fitness value, as determined by an evaluation function, increases the probability that individual solutions are mutated and reproduced. After several generations (i.e. iterations of the process), the population converges to one or several local maxima. Pseudocode for the basic procedure is shown in Fig. 5.2.

The major differences to genetic algorithms [114] that were employed previously for model matching by Hill et al. [110] are listed below: First, solutions are not required to be encoded as bit-strings in artificial chromosomes but are stored as real-valued vectors. Second, there is no cross-over operator for mutation (recombination) and no bit-inversion. Instead, solutions are modified by adding a random vector from a multivariate zero-mean Gaussian distribution.

### 5.2.1 Evolutionary algorithm

One individual in the population of solutions represents one possible shape configuration, consisting of a similarity transform and $c$ shape parameters. For initialization, all shape parameters $y_m$ are randomized according to their variance $\lambda_m$. The pose parameters (translation, rotation, scale) are estimated from the respective mean values of the training samples (using

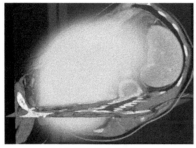 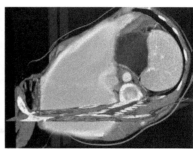

**(a)** Initial distribution          **(b)** After converged search

**Figure 5.3:** Shape population in an image after initialization (a) and after convergence (b). All shapes are rendered as transparent solids, overlap increases the density color-coded from light to dark. While the left population is spread widely and only appears as a diffuse cloud, the right population is centered closely around the final solution. Both images display 5000 individual shapes.

relative coordinates for location[1]) and are also randomized using a Gaussian distribution.

To evaluate the fitness $w_s$ of an individual solution $s$, the probabilities $p_b^{(i)}$ that a landmark $i$ is part of the true boundary are estimated for all landmarks and are multiplied. Written in exponential form, this results in:

$$w_s = \exp\left(\frac{v}{n} \sum_i \log p_b^{(i)}\right) \tag{5.1}$$

Here, $n$ holds the number of employed appearance models and $v$ is a constant that determines the speed of convergence of the search process. Chosing larger values for $v$ amplifies the probability differences between different solutions and thus influences the amount of well-fitting solutions which is selected in the following step. While the particle filtering method used by de Bruijne and Nielsen [62] requires all $p_b^{(i)}$ to express the likelihood of a boundary at this position, the scheme presented in this thesis does not have these strict constraints. In fact, if using one of the non-linear appearance models with kNN-classifier from Sec. 4.1, the calculated $p_b^{(i)}$ will express the posterior probability of a boundary, and thus, the fitness func-

---

[1]Coordinates are expressed relative to image boundaries, i.e. $(0.5, 0.5, 0.5)$ corresponds to the center of a volume.

tion in Eq. 5.1 directly expresses the statistical evidence for the individual shape in the image.

Having evaluated the fitness $w_s$ for all individuals $s$ in the current population, a selection step choses the solutions that are going to evolve for the next iteration. The selection process is implemented as a random sampling in which each individual $s$ gets a chance of reproduction proportional to its fitness $w_s$. Subsequently, all drawn individuals are mutated with the current standard deviation $\sigma_t$. More explicitly, all shape parameters $y_m$ are perturbed by a random value from the Gaussian distribution $(0, \sigma_t \sqrt{\lambda_m})$, the scale factor is perturbed by a random distribution $(0, \sigma_t \sigma_{scale})$, and similar for rotation and translation parameters. While all $\lambda_m$, being the eigenvalues of the SSM, are known, the other parameters $\sigma_{scale}$, $\sigma_{rot}$ and $\sigma_{trans}$ are generally unknown and must be estimated.

For the following iteration $t + 1$, the common standard deviation is reduced using $\sigma_{t+1} = \sigma \sigma_t$ (with $0 < \sigma < 1$). Typical values for $\sigma$ are 0.8 to 0.95. This corresponds to a reduction in step size of the optimizer and enables us to use a relatively large $\sigma_0$ to conduct an exhaustive search in the beginning and still obtain a stable convergence towards the end. After a fixed number of x iterations, optimization is stopped. If x is large enough, most individuals will have converged towards the same point (Fig. 5.3). The individual reaching the maximum fitness during evolution is the final solution.

### 5.2.2 Landmark reduction

In the presented segmentation scheme, the evolutionary algorithm is run to find a rough initialization in a strongly down-sampled version of the image. For this purpose, a simplified version of the SSM (i.e. with fewer landmarks) is equally suitable, and considerably faster during the search. The process of choosing the best landmarks for the reduced model is essentially a mesh simplification problem. There is a priority queue of landmarks to be eliminated which is sorted according to the performance indices $\xi$ (from Eq. 4.8) of the corresponding appearance models. However, landmarks cannot always be removed from that queue in their given order, as that may leave certain parts of the surface completely empty, and the reduced landmark set must still cover all parts of the surface. Therefore, a constraint is introduced which ensures that a landmark cannot be deleted if the resulting gap would be larger than a certain geodesic radius r, which is estimated by the number of traversed edges in the SSM. For $r = 1$, this means there

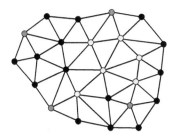

**Figure 5.4:** Example for a landmark reduction process with maximum gap radius $r = 1$. The black dots have been deleted from the mesh, the red ones cannot be deleted because they are the only remaining neighbors of at least one removed vertex. The green dots can still be deleted, and will be removed with a priority deduced from the corresponding appearance model performance.

must exist at least one "surviving" landmark in the direct neighborhood of each deleted one – see Fig. 5.4 for a small example.

The landmark reduction procedure is implemented as a greedy algorithm as suggested for mesh decimation by Kobbelt et al. [134]. Depending on the number of landmarks in the original SSM, a maximum gap radius of $r = 1$ or 2 delivers good results. Figure 5.5 shows the result of a decimated SSM of the liver.

## 5.3 Local search

Once a rough initial transform for the SSM is determined, a local optimization algorithm adapts the model further to the data and delivers the final segmentation. Since from experience, the available training data is rarely sufficient to reach an acceptable generalization ability of the SSM, the developed method allows for additional flexibility during the search, following the approaches described in Sec. 2.6.5. Basis of the method is a deformable surface model defined as a triangulated mesh $M = (V, E)$ with vertices $p, q \in V$ and edges $[p, q] \in E$. M has the same topology as the associated statistical shape model, where for each vertex p in the mesh, there is a corresponding vertex $\tilde{p}$ in the SSM. The evolution of the deformable model is controlled by the Lagrangian equation of motion: at every vertex $p_i$, a regularizing internal force $F_{int}(p_i)$ and a data-driven external force $F_{ext}(p_i)$

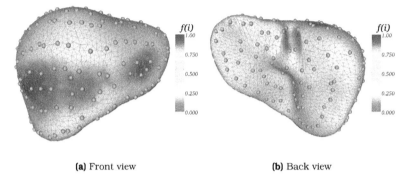

(a) Front view          (b) Back view

**Figure 5.5:** Reduced set of landmarks on a shape model of the liver. The performance $\xi$ of the local appearance models is color-coded over the entire surface. The full set of landmarks is displayed using a triangular grid, the reduced set is shown as small spheres. The maximum gap radius r is 2. It is clearly visible how landmarks evade the low-performance sections of the surface by grouping around them.

are applied[2]. In discrete form, this can be written as:

$$p_i^{t+1} = p_i^t + F_{int}(p_i^t) + F_{ext}(p_i^t) \tag{5.2}$$

In the following, the derivations for both internal and external forces will be presented in detail.

### 5.3.1 Internal forces

The task of the internal forces is to keep the shape of the deformable surface similar to the one of the template defined by the underlying shape model. Section 5.3.4 explains how to determine the parameters for the SSM for a given deformable model during evolution. Here, it is assumed that the ideal shape template is known.

Most important in this context is the local similarity, where the relative locations of neighboring vertices do not deviate too much from the template.

---

[2]Technically, $F_{int}(p_i)$ and $F_{ext}(p_i)$ are impulses. However, nomenclature of image analysis is followed here, which traditionally denotes these terms as "forces" [171].

Kaus et al. [127] chose the differences in edge length as the driving force of the internal energy. However, this is only one part of local similarity. The other part, values of angles between neighboring faces, is also important. These two ingredients correspond to the concepts of tension and rigidity which are also used to define the internal energy of a snake [125]. When defining the internal forces, Newton's Third Law of Motion has to be obeyed: for every action, there is an equal and opposite reaction. This means that internal forces may not alter the overall position of the deformable surface, as in all internal forces must sum up to zero.

To implement tension forces, every edge $[p, q]$ is modeled as a linear spring with neutral length $|\tilde{p} - \tilde{q}|$, which is the length of $[p, q]$ in the template. Consequently, the tension force on a vertex $p$ in the direction towards $q$ is:

$$F_T(p, q) = \alpha \left( |p - q| - |\tilde{p} - \tilde{q}| \right) \frac{p - q}{|p - q|} \tag{5.3}$$

where $\alpha$ defines the strength of the tension force and is constant for all $[p, q] \in E$. Thus, the total tension force for a vertex is the sum over the forces along all of its edges:

$$F_T(p) = \sum_{[p,q] \in E} F_T(p, q) \tag{5.4}$$

Rigidity forces are modeled as linear springs along the angle $\theta$ between two faces: for every edge $[p_1, p_2] \in E$, adjacent triangles $[p_1, p_2, q_1]$ and $[p_2, p_1, q_2]$ form an angle $\theta$ that strives towards the corresponding angle $\tilde{\theta}$ in the SSM. Here, $q_1, q_2$ are called the outer vertices of $[p_1, p_2]$, and both together form the set $V_O([p_1, p_2])$. Figure 5.6 gives an overview over the constellation.

The rigidity force for an outer vertex $q \in V_O([p_1, p_2])$ is calculated using a rotation:

$$F_R(q, [p_1, p_2]) = T(q, [p_1, p_2], \beta\delta)) - q \tag{5.5}$$

where $T(q, [p_1, p_2], x)$ is a rotation of point $q$ around the edge $[p_1, p_2]$ by $x$ degrees, and $\beta$ is the strength of the rigidity force. To define $\delta$ for both outer vertices, let us consider the case of a constellation where distances $d_1$ and $d_2$ are different from each other. In order to move both $q_1$ and $q_2$ over the same distance, the outer vertex that is further away requires a smaller rotation angle due to the leverage effect:

$$\delta = \frac{d_{op}}{d_1 + d_2} \left( \theta - \tilde{\theta} \right) \tag{5.6}$$

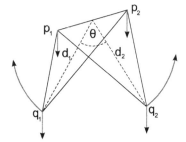

**Figure 5.6:** Two adjacent triangles form the angle θ. Internal rigidity forces striving for a larger angle directly affect the outer vertices $q_1$ and $q_2$ (red arrows), but also the edge vertices $p_1$ and $p_2$ to maintain the equilibrium of the constellation (green arrows).

where $d_{op}$ is the distance to the opposing outer vertex (i.e. $d_2$ when calculating δ for $q_1$ and vice versa). To maintain the equilibrium required by Newton's Third Law of Motion, forces on $q_1$ and $q_2$ must be neutralized within the constellation. The neutralizing forces act equally on all four vertices of a constellation and are defined as:

$$F_N([p_1,p_2]) = -\frac{1}{4}(F_R(q_1, [p_1,p_2]) + F_R(q_2, [p_1,p_2])) \tag{5.7}$$

Overall, this results in a total rigidity force of:

$$F_R(p) = \sum_{[p_1,p_2]\in E} \begin{cases} F_R(p, [p_1,p_2]) + F_N([p_1,p_2]) & \text{if } p \in V_O([p_1,p_2]) \\ F_N([p_1,p_2]) & \text{if } p = p_1 \lor p = p_2 \\ \vec{0} & \text{else} \end{cases} \tag{5.8}$$

Finally, the internal force for a given vertex is the sum of tension force and rigidity force:

$$F_{int}(p) = F_T(p) + F_R(p) \tag{5.9}$$

### 5.3.2 External forces

The external forces drive the deformable surface towards the best fit to the data. As in the ASM search procedure, the goodness of fit is evaluated for all $p \in V$ at $p$ itself and additional at $K$ positions on each side of the surface. This procedure leads to $2K + 1$ probes for each vertex, enumerated

as $k \in [-K..K]$, and all spaced with a distance of $d_P$ along the normal vector $\vec{n}(p)$. A linear spring force then drives the vertex in the direction of the optimal position $s(p)$:

$$F_{ext}(p) = \gamma(s(p) - p) \tag{5.10}$$

where $\gamma$ is the strength of the external forces. In past work, $s(p)$ has always been determined independently for each vertex $p$, generally by:

$$s(p) = p + \vec{n}(p) \operatorname*{argmax}_{k} p(g_k|model) \tag{5.11}$$

This procedure is suboptimal, because it uses merely one evaluation result from all performed probes (the maximum value) – all others are neglected. Thus, it usually produces a considerable amount of outliers. While one can argue that outlier removal should be accomplished by the internal forces, these do not have any information about the other probe results and thus cannot chose appropriate alternatives for $s(p)$. For this reason, the external forces should draw the vertices to a smooth and outlier-free new configuration. Thus the best fit to the data is defined as the configuration of vertices that minimizes the sum of individual costs of fit given a hard constraint on the maximum deviation between neighboring vertices. The following section details how this configuration can be efficiently determined.

### 5.3.3 Optimal surface detection

Detecting optimal surfaces in volumetric data is a frequent problem in segmentation with deformable models. While the 2D analogue (the detection of an optimal path in an image) can be solved efficiently using dynamic programming techniques, no computationally tractable method for the 3D case was known until recently. Then, Wu and Chen presented a method to transform the problem into that of finding the minimum s-t cut in a graph [263], which can be solved in polynomial time. The method was later evaluated especially for the segmentation of volumetric image data [154]. The authors presume that the surface to be detected is terrain-like, i.e. that it intersects all columns of a given volume at the optimal locations. If this is true, the algorithm finds the global optimum given hard constraints on the smoothness of the surface, which are defined as the maximum steepness between neighboring columns. They also use this method to detect cylindrical surfaces by unrolling them to a terrain-like structure. In a later publication [151], they presented an extension for closed surfaces. In the

following, the algorithm for terrain-like surfaces is reviewed and a solution to apply it to closed triangular surfaces (as the deformable model used in this work) is presented.

The first step is to build a directed graph $G = (N, D)$ from the volume the surface should pass through. For each voxel in the volume of size $(X, Y, Z)$, one node $n(x, y, z) \in N$ is created. For each column $(x, y)$ in the graph (without loss of generality assuming that columns are oriented along the z-axis), directed edges with infinite weight are added from $n(x, y, z)$ to $n(x, y, z - 1)$ for $z > 0$. Subsequently, directed edges with infinite weight are added between neighboring columns $col(x_1, y_1)$ and $col(x_2, y_2)$ (directly adjacent in x- or y-direction) from $n_1(x_1, y_1, z)$ to $n_2(x_2, y_2, \max(0, z - \Delta))$. $\Delta$ is the maximum steepness between neighboring vertices and implements the smoothness constraint.

Assume that the fitting costs for the surface at voxel $(x, y, z)$ are stored in $f(x, y, z)$. Then a weight is computed for each $n(x, y, z) \in N$ according to:

$$w(x, y, z) = \begin{cases} f(x, y, z) & \text{for } z = 0 \\ f(x, y, z) - f(x, y, z - 1) & \text{for } z > 0 \end{cases} \tag{5.12}$$

Before running the s-t cut algorithm, an additional source node $n_s$ and a sink node $n_t$ are added to the graph. All previously inserted nodes are connected to these two in the following way: every node with $w(x, y, z) \geq 0$ is connected to $n_t$ by a directed edge of weight $w(x, y, z)$, and $n_s$ is connected to every node with $w(x, y, z) < 0$ by a directed edge of weight $-w(x, y, z)$. Employing an s-t cut algorithm like the one presented in [18], the graph can now be divided into a source set S with $n_s \in S$ and sink set T with $n_t \in T$. The optimal intersection point for each column is the node $n(x, y, z) \in S$ with the largest z-coordinate.

The extension of this algorithm to closed surfaces $M = (V, E)$ is straightforward: the new columns in the graph are defined as a series of $2K + 1$ probes along the normal vector at each vertex $p \in V$. These probes are ordered from inside to outside of the surface with $-K \leq k \leq K$ and inserted into the graph as $n(p, k)$. The edges connecting all nodes of a column $(p)$ are then inserted as described above. Next, directed edges between neighboring columns $col(p_1)$ and $col(p_2)$ are added from $n(p_1, k)$ to $n(p_2, \max(0, k - \Delta))$. $col(p_1)$ and $col(p_2)$ count as adjacent if $[p_1, p_2] \in E$ (Fig. 5.7). Replacing the fitting costs $f(x, y, z)$ by $f(p, k)$, the addition of source and sink nodes to the graph is performed as in the terrain-like case. After the s-t cut, the optimal displacements $k_{opt}(p)$ are given by the largest k with $n(p, k) \in S$.

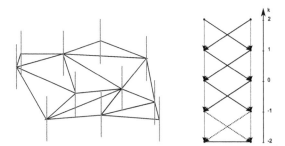

**Figure 5.7:** Optimal surface detection for closed triangle meshes: On the left, a section of the mesh is displayed; the different probe positions for each vertex are displayed by a green line. The right side illustrates how two adjacent probe lines are represented in the graph (here for $K = 2$ and $\Delta = 1$). All edges have infinite weight, the dotted connections are optional.

### 5.3.4 Model search scheme

To increase robustness of the deformable model, external forces are calculated using a multi-resolution approach. The image volume to be analyzed is down-sampled to $N_R - 1$ smaller scales, forming an image pyramid of size $N_R$. For each down-sampling step, the image is first smoothed with a Gaussian filter and then resampled to half the previous resolution in each direction $x, y, z$. Resolution $R_0$ corresponds to the original image, $R_1$ is down-sampled once, $R_2$ is down-sampled twice, and so on. Since external forces are based on the best fit of local appearance models as described in Sec. 4.1, these models have to be trained for multiple resolutions, too. In case of profile models, the spacing between two adjacent points in a profile $g$ is doubled with each down-sampling step to capture a wider range of image information in lower resolutions. During model deformation, distances $d_P$ between two adjacent probes along the normal vector of a vertex $p$ follow the same logic and are doubled at each resolution change to achieve a larger search radius.

The optimal surface detection algorithm described above delivers the optimal displacements $k_{opt}(p)$ for all $p \in V$. Thus, the optimal positions are defined as:

$$s(p) = p + \vec{n}(p)k_{opt}(p) \tag{5.13}$$

with $\vec{n}(p)$ as the normal vector for $p$. The gained coordinates $s(p)$ form the basis of the external forces from Eq. 5.10. In addition, they are used to

determine the parameters of the underlying shape model, which consist of a similarity transform to the image volume (i.e. the pose) and the actual shape parameters $y_m$. Shape and pose are determined by the same procedure as presented by Cootes et al. [43] for the Active Shape Model algorithm. First, the best pose $\mathbf{T}$ is determined using a Procrustes matching of the current model to the new coordinates. Then, the shape vector can be calculated by:

$$\mathbf{y} = \mathbf{P}^{-1}(\mathbf{x} - \bar{\mathbf{x}}) \qquad (5.14)$$

with $\mathbf{P} = (p_1|p_2|\ldots|p_c)$ as the matrix of eigenvectors and $\mathbf{x}$ as the concatenation of $s(p)$ transformed into model space by $\mathbf{T}^{-1}$ (refer to Sec. 2.6.2 for a more detailed description of the ASM approach). Although it is possible to update external forces and SSM at every deformation step of the surface, this procedure is impractical from a computational point of view. In practice, an update every $N_u$ iterations is sufficient – for all experiments in this thesis, $N_u$ was set to 10.

## 5.4 Appearance model weighting

A common variant for model-based search algorithms are weighting schemes, which means that different landmarks have varying influence on the model evolution. Typically, weighting is employed to reduce the influence of outliers in the segmentation process. Due to utilizing the optimal surface detection, the effect of outliers is greatly reduced in this work, but there might still be a possibility for improvement: the key idea is to use the performance indices $\xi$ from Eq. 4.8 to weight the fitting costs individually for each landmark.

Given that the optimal surface detection finds the globally best solution within the given constraints, it is sufficient to multiply the fitting costs $c_f^{(i)}$, delivered by appearance model $i$ at the current position, with the corresponding $\xi^{(i)}$. The resulting value is then used to determine the weights for the surface detection as described by Eq. 5.12. A prerequisite for this procedure is that all fitting costs $c_f^{(i)}$ deliver values in the same interval, which is assured by normalizing all appearance models (Sec. 4.3.2).

## 5.5 Performance measures

According to a survey on evaluation methods for image segmentation by Zhang [269], there are three major approaches to evaluate the performance of segmentation algorithms: the analytical, the empirical goodness and the empirical discrepancy approach. The first one is mainly of theoretical nature, and the second one follows rather general criteria (e.g. a segmented region should be smooth and homogeneous). The third approach, which is followed here, consists of a comparison of the segmentation to be evaluated with a corresponding reference. Since segmented images are required for training the statistical models anyway, this procedure is best conducted using cross-validation.

There exists a whole variety of comparison metrics between images, as the ones presented by Niessen et al. [176] and Gerig et al. [91]. For the experiments in this thesis, the following five measures are used: volumetric overlap error, relative volumetric difference, average surface distance, RMS surface distance and maximum surface distance.

There are several variants of the volumetric overlap, the one used here is commonly named Tanimoto- or Jaccard-coefficient. Given two regions A and B, it is defined as:

$$C_T = \frac{|A \cap B|}{|A \cup B|} \tag{5.15}$$

where $|.|$ denotes the volume of a region. This coefficient yields 1 if both shapes are identical and 0 for no overlap at all. To transform the measure into an error metric, the obvious way is to negate it. Thus, the volumetric overlap error is defined as:

$$\text{VOE} = 1 - C_T \tag{5.16}$$

The VOE allows a good estimate how much a segmentation is in accordance with a reference, but it does not reveal if deviations are mainly caused by over- or under-segmentation of the object of interest. For this reason, the relative volumetric difference is calculated, specified as:

$$\text{RVD} = \frac{|A| - |B|}{|B|} \tag{5.17}$$

assuming the B is the reference. The RVD yields 0 if the two segmentations have exactly the same value, otherwise a positive or negative value. Note

that even if the result is 0, that does not imply that both segmentations actually overlap – they could be at completely different locations in the image. For this reason, the RVD is no metric, but together with the volumetric overlap error it is still useful to estimate segmentation accuracy.

The remaining three measures are based on surface distances. The concept of surface distances is the logical extension of the well-known point-to-surface distances, which are defined (from a point x to a surface Y) as:

$$d(x, Y) = \min_{y \in Y} \|x - y\| \qquad (5.18)$$

where $\|.\|$ denotes the Euclidean distance. When defining surface distances, symmetry as a precondition for every metric has to be ensured. Thus, the average surface distance is defined as:

$$ASD(X, Y) = \frac{1}{|X| + |Y|} \left( \int_{x \in X} d(x, Y) dx + \int_{y \in Y} d(y, X) dy \right) \qquad (5.19)$$

where $|.|$ denotes the area of a surface. In a similar fashion, the root mean squared surface distance (equivalent to the RMS error) is defined as:

$$RMSSD(X, Y) = \frac{1}{|X| + |Y|} \sqrt{\int_{x \in X} d^2(x, Y) dx + \int_{y \in Y} d^2(y, X) dy} \qquad (5.20)$$

Finally, the maximum surface distance is given by:

$$MSD(X, Y) = \max \left\{ \max_{x \in X} d(x, Y), \max_{y \in Y} d(y, X) \right\} \qquad (5.21)$$

Taken together, these five measures should be able to provide a good estimate relating to the performance of the proposed segmentation algorithm.

# 6 Experiments and Results

*"Data, data, data!" he cried impatiently.
"I can't make bricks without clay."*

— *Sir Arthur Conan Doyle, "Sherlock Holmes:
the Adventure of the Copper Beeches" (1892)*

In this chapter, the developed segmentation approach – comprised of statistical shape model, statistical appearance model and search algorithm – is
evaluated on three clinical applications. To show the general applicability of
the method, three different modalities were chosen for the tests: Computed
Tomography (CT), Magnetic Resonance Imaging (MRI), and Ultrasound (US).
All modalities deliver full 3D volumes of varying voxel resolution. In addition to the different modalities, the three chosen objects of interest also
exhibit different characteristics with respect to their shape. The liver, examined in Sec. 6.1, features an extremely high variability from person to
person and should pose a strong challenge to shape modeling. The left lobe
of the lung, treated in Sec. 6.2, is more uniform over the population, but
varies considerably over time during the breathing cycle. The last object
of interest considered is the prostate (Sec. 6.3) – in comparison to the two
other organs, its shape is fairly stable, but its small size and the noisy US
modality used for acquisition make it a challenging target for image analysis nonetheless.

## 6.1 Evaluation on the liver (CT)

Main motivation to apply the developed algorithms to the liver is a project
for surgery planning [168]. To calculate and visualize the optimal resection
strategy for liver tumors, the liver tissue, vessel systems, and tumors have
to be segmented beforehand. Performed manually, segmentation of the liver
tissue takes 30 to 45 minutes and is the most time-consuming section of
the planning process (all other steps sum up to approximately 20 minutes).

7

Therefore, an automated solution for this task would speed up the planning process considerably and make it available for a larger number of patients.

### 6.1.1 Data material

The used liver images were acquired on a variety of CT scanners from different manufacturers, some with 4 detector rows, others with 16 or 64 rows. Consequently, the voxel spacing varies considerable: The in-plane spacing lies between 0.55 and 0.8 mm, the inter-slice distance between 1 and 3 mm. There is no overlap between neighboring slices. To smooth the data, anisotropic diffusion filtering [188] was used as a preprocessing step for all image volumes. The filter was run over 20 iterations, using a timestep of 0.05 and a conductance of 2.5. For this experiment, a total of 45 volumes were utilized. Most of them are pathologic and include tumors, metastases and cysts of different sizes. The huge variety of shapes is displayed in Fig. 6.1. The reference segmentations for training were created manually by radiological experts, working slice-by-slice in transversal view. They are defined as the entire liver tissue including all internal structures such as vessel systems, tumors etc. In general, a vessel counts as internal if it is completely surrounded by liver tissue (in the transversal view). The large vessels that enter the liver (*Vena Cava* and portal vein) were segmented in the part which is enclosed by liver tissue, i.e. as the convex hull of the liver shape in that area.

### 6.1.2 Shape model construction

After converting the manual segmentations to meshes using the methods from Sec. 3.1, the point correspondences were determined over all 45 shapes. Three different strategies were used to build the model, each time with 2562 landmarks (created by 4 subdivisions of the icosahedron). First, the gradient-based optimization presented in Sec. 3.3 was run, which resulted in the first model. The resulting landmarks were then reconfigured using the technique from Sec. 3.4 to reach an equally dense distribution over the entire surface, yielding the second model. For the third model, the reconfiguration step was employed continuously during the optimization, i.e. every 10 iterations. On a standard desktop PC, the computations took approximately 30 hours for the first model and 50 hours including the continuous reconfiguration.

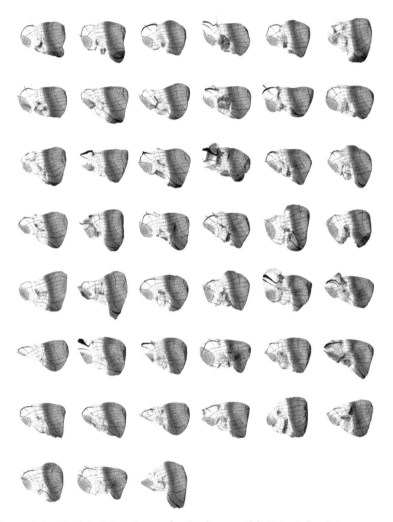

**Figure 6.1:** All 45 training shapes for the liver model. Detected point correspondences are visualized using a color-coded coordinate grid.

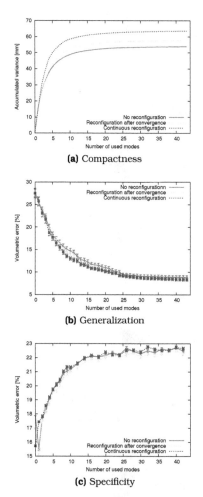

(a) Compactness

(b) Generalization

(c) Specificity

**Figure 6.2:** Quantitative comparison between three different optimization approaches for the liver model.

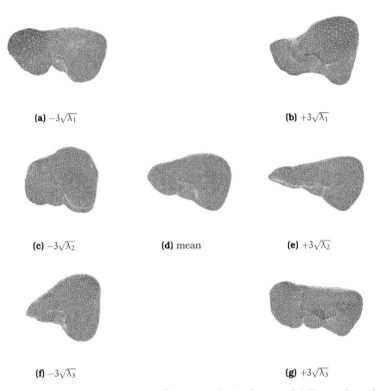

(a) $-3\sqrt{\lambda_1}$               (b) $+3\sqrt{\lambda_1}$

(c) $-3\sqrt{\lambda_2}$      (d) mean      (e) $+3\sqrt{\lambda_2}$

(f) $-3\sqrt{\lambda_3}$               (g) $+3\sqrt{\lambda_3}$

**Figure 6.3:** The three largest modes of variation for the liver model. For each mode, the shapes three standard deviations away from the mean are shown.

All created models were evaluated using the modified generalization and specificity measures from Sec. 3.5. For completeness, the compactness of the models was also calculated. The resulting graphs are shown in Fig. 6.2.

For a qualitative inspection of correspondences (for the model built with the third strategy), a color-coded spherical coordinate grid is laid over the training shapes in Fig. 6.1. Additionally, the three largest modes of variation detected in the training set are displayed in Fig. 6.3.

### 6.1.3 Appearance models

For the evaluation of appearance models, five images were randomly selected and excluded from training. A number of appearance models from Sec. 4.1 were built with different parameters for the original image resolution and four down-sampled versions. First, Gaussian intensity and gradient profiles were build in normalized and unnormalized versions of 3, 5, 7 and 9 samples length. In accordance with the voxel spacing of the training images, spacing between two consecutive profile points was set to 1 mm (in the original resolution). Subsequently, non-linear (kNN) intensity and gradient profiles were constructed of the same lengths, again normalized and unnormalized. Finally, histogram region models with 8, 16 and 32 bins per histogram were built for regions of 7, 11 and 15 cube voxels each. All models were evaluated using the simulated search from Sec. 4.3 on the five excluded images. Results are listed for each resolution in Table 6.1, a compressed presentation using box-plots is given in Fig. 6.4.

The best-performing appearance model – in this case the 5 samples long normalized intensity profile with kNN classifier – was selected for the clustering step from Sec. 4.2. Using varying sizes for the mean-shift kernel and specified minimum cluster sizes, four different clustered appearance models were generated: The first model combined the 2562 landmark models to 432 clusters, the second one to 44 clusters, the third to 7 clusters and the fourth model pooled all individual models into one general appearance model. As the clustering leads to a higher density of samples in the space where the kNN-classfier is operating, the appearance model was also clustered with the next-higher number of samples (i.e. the 7 samples long normalized intensity profile). In this case, the clustering lead to models consisting of 424, 44, 6 and one cluster. The performance of the clustered appearance models was evaluated as described above and added to Table 6.1 and Fig. 6.4. Overall, the 7 samples long normalized intensity profile using a kNN classifer working on the data clustered with strategy 3 (i.e. 6

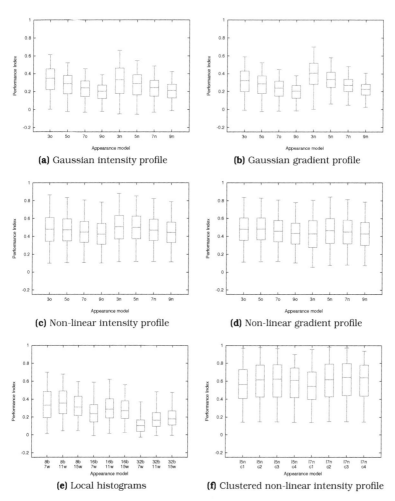

(a) Gaussian intensity profile

(b) Gaussian gradient profile

(c) Non-linear intensity profile

(d) Non-linear gradient profile

(e) Local histograms

(f) Clustered non-linear intensity profile

**Figure 6.4:** Performance of different appearance models on liver CT images. Box-plots show median and surrounding quartiles of calculated performance index over all landmarks and all resolutions. Whiskers indicate the 5% and 95% quantiles. Profile models are labeled by their length, followed by an 'o' for original values or 'n' for normalized values. The histogram models are labeled by their number of bins ('b') and the width of the region they are collected in ('w'). For the clustered models, the clustering strategy is given as c1 to c4 – see the text for details.

clusters) delivered the best results with an average performance index of 0.61.

### 6.1.4 Segmentation results

To evaluate the automated segmentation approach, cross-validation was employed and 9 sets of images were generated, with 5 images left out each time. For each set, a specific shape and appearance model was constructed. All shape models are based on correspondences determined by the initial optimization using continuous landmark reconfiguration. The employed appearance models are the clustered versions of the 7 samples long normalized non-linear intensity profiles.

#### Initialization

The first step for the automatic initialization required the generation of a reduced set of landmarks, as described in Sec. 5.2.2. The geodesic radius in which a landmark must exist was set to $r = 2$, which resulted in a decimation to 215 landmarks. Global search was conducted with the genetic algorithm from Sec. 5.2.1, which was run on the 4 times down-sampled image to provide the largest possible capture range. From preliminary tests, the following set of parameters for the algorithm was considered as viable: 10 shape parameters to optimize, using a population of 1000 individuals over $x = 40$ iterations, starting with a perturbation factor of $\sigma_0 = 0.4$ and ending at $\sigma_{40} = 0.05$ (which corresponds to $\sigma = 0.95$). The speed of convergence was set to $v = 5$ and the perturbation factor for translation was set to $\sigma_{trans} = 20$.

To evaluate the dependency of the genetic algorithm on these parameters, several series of global search were conducted. For each series, one parameter was modified within a certain range and the algorithm was run on the first test set, consisting of five random images. As some of the considered parameters influence each other, the following rules were applied to minimize interference: when modifying the number of iterations $x$, $\sigma$ was modified too, in order to ensure that $\sigma_x$ used during the last iteration always remained same value. For the same reason, $\sigma$ was also adjusted when modifying the initial perturbation factor $\sigma_0$.

As a measure of success of the search, the volumetric overlap between the found solution and corresponding reference segmentation was calculated. In Fig. 6.5, results are displayed as graphs over the varying parameter.

| App-Model | $R_0$ | $R_1$ | $R_2$ | $R_3$ | $R_4$ | Average |
|---|---|---|---|---|---|---|
| Gauss-IP3o | 0.24 ± 0.14 | 0.32 ± 0.15 | 0.37 ± 0.16 | 0.36 ± 0.17 | 0.37 ± 0.14 | 0.33 ± 0.15 |
| Gauss-IP5o | 0.19 ± 0.12 | 0.26 ± 0.14 | 0.30 ± 0.15 | 0.29 ± 0.14 | 0.33 ± 0.12 | 0.27 ± 0.14 |
| Gauss-IP7o | 0.15 ± 0.11 | 0.22 ± 0.12 | 0.25 ± 0.13 | 0.24 ± 0.12 | 0.28 ± 0.11 | 0.23 ± 0.12 |
| Gauss-IP9o | 0.12 ± 0.09 | 0.19 ± 0.10 | 0.21 ± 0.11 | 0.21 ± 0.10 | 0.24 ± 0.10 | 0.19 ± 0.10 |
| Gauss-IP3n | 0.19 ± 0.16 | 0.29 ± 0.18 | 0.36 ± 0.20 | 0.36 ± 0.21 | 0.39 ± 0.16 | 0.32 ± 0.18 |
| Gauss-IP5n | 0.16 ± 0.14 | 0.25 ± 0.15 | 0.29 ± 0.15 | 0.30 ± 0.16 | 0.35 ± 0.14 | 0.27 ± 0.15 |
| Gauss-IP7n | 0.14 ± 0.11 | 0.22 ± 0.11 | 0.25 ± 0.13 | 0.25 ± 0.13 | 0.31 ± 0.13 | 0.23 ± 0.12 |
| Gauss-IP9n | 0.12 ± 0.09 | 0.19 ± 0.10 | 0.22 ± 0.11 | 0.22 ± 0.11 | 0.26 ± 0.13 | 0.20 ± 0.11 |
| Gauss-GP3o | 0.22 ± 0.14 | 0.31 ± 0.15 | 0.35 ± 0.16 | 0.32 ± 0.16 | 0.36 ± 0.14 | 0.31 ± 0.15 |
| Gauss-GP5o | 0.20 ± 0.13 | 0.28 ± 0.13 | 0.30 ± 0.14 | 0.27 ± 0.14 | 0.32 ± 0.13 | 0.27 ± 0.14 |
| Gauss-GP7o | 0.16 ± 0.11 | 0.24 ± 0.11 | 0.25 ± 0.12 | 0.24 ± 0.11 | 0.27 ± 0.12 | 0.23 ± 0.12 |
| Gauss-GP9o | 0.14 ± 0.09 | 0.20 ± 0.10 | 0.20 ± 0.11 | 0.21 ± 0.10 | 0.23 ± 0.10 | 0.19 ± 0.10 |
| Gauss-GP3n | 0.29 ± 0.17 | 0.41 ± 0.17 | 0.46 ± 0.17 | 0.40 ± 0.17 | 0.41 ± 0.16 | 0.39 ± 0.17 |
| Gauss-GP5n | 0.25 ± 0.12 | 0.34 ± 0.12 | 0.36 ± 0.12 | 0.34 ± 0.12 | 0.36 ± 0.14 | 0.33 ± 0.12 |
| Gauss-GP7n | 0.20 ± 0.10 | 0.27 ± 0.10 | 0.28 ± 0.10 | 0.28 ± 0.11 | 0.30 ± 0.12 | 0.27 ± 0.10 |
| Gauss-GP9n | 0.16 ± 0.08 | 0.22 ± 0.08 | 0.23 ± 0.08 | 0.23 ± 0.10 | 0.26 ± 0.11 | 0.22 ± 0.09 |
| kNN-IP3o | 0.29 ± 0.13 | 0.45 ± 0.15 | 0.54 ± 0.18 | 0.55 ± 0.18 | 0.57 ± 0.17 | 0.48 ± 0.16 |
| kNN-IP5o | 0.30 ± 0.13 | 0.45 ± 0.15 | 0.53 ± 0.17 | 0.54 ± 0.18 | 0.54 ± 0.17 | 0.47 ± 0.16 |
| kNN-IP7o | 0.30 ± 0.13 | 0.45 ± 0.14 | 0.51 ± 0.16 | 0.50 ± 0.17 | 0.51 ± 0.18 | 0.45 ± 0.16 |
| kNN-IP9o | 0.30 ± 0.13 | 0.43 ± 0.14 | 0.48 ± 0.16 | 0.46 ± 0.17 | 0.48 ± 0.18 | 0.43 ± 0.16 |
| kNN-IP3n | 0.31 ± 0.14 | 0.48 ± 0.16 | 0.57 ± 0.17 | 0.57 ± 0.18 | 0.58 ± 0.17 | 0.50 ± 0.17 |
| kNN-IP5n | 0.32 ± 0.14 | 0.49 ± 0.16 | 0.57 ± 0.17 | 0.55 ± 0.17 | 0.55 ± 0.17 | 0.50 ± 0.16 |
| kNN-IP7n | 0.32 ± 0.14 | 0.47 ± 0.15 | 0.53 ± 0.16 | 0.51 ± 0.17 | 0.52 ± 0.18 | 0.47 ± 0.16 |
| kNN-IP9n | 0.33 ± 0.14 | 0.46 ± 0.15 | 0.49 ± 0.16 | 0.47 ± 0.16 | 0.49 ± 0.18 | 0.45 ± 0.16 |
| kNN-GP3o | 0.32 ± 0.14 | 0.47 ± 0.15 | 0.54 ± 0.16 | 0.52 ± 0.18 | 0.54 ± 0.18 | 0.48 ± 0.16 |
| kNN-GP5o | 0.33 ± 0.14 | 0.48 ± 0.15 | 0.54 ± 0.16 | 0.52 ± 0.18 | 0.54 ± 0.18 | 0.48 ± 0.16 |
| kNN-GP7o | 0.33 ± 0.14 | 0.47 ± 0.15 | 0.50 ± 0.16 | 0.48 ± 0.17 | 0.51 ± 0.19 | 0.46 ± 0.16 |
| kNN-GP9o | 0.33 ± 0.14 | 0.45 ± 0.15 | 0.47 ± 0.16 | 0.45 ± 0.18 | 0.48 ± 0.19 | 0.43 ± 0.16 |
| kNN-GP3n | 0.26 ± 0.16 | 0.44 ± 0.18 | 0.52 ± 0.18 | 0.44 ± 0.20 | 0.47 ± 0.18 | 0.43 ± 0.18 |
| kNN-GP5n | 0.29 ± 0.16 | 0.48 ± 0.18 | 0.55 ± 0.18 | 0.48 ± 0.19 | 0.51 ± 0.18 | 0.46 ± 0.18 |
| kNN-GP7n | 0.30 ± 0.16 | 0.48 ± 0.17 | 0.51 ± 0.17 | 0.46 ± 0.19 | 0.49 ± 0.19 | 0.45 ± 0.18 |
| kNN-GP9n | 0.30 ± 0.16 | 0.46 ± 0.17 | 0.47 ± 0.17 | 0.44 ± 0.18 | 0.47 ± 0.19 | 0.43 ± 0.17 |
| H08b-07w | 0.16 ± 0.11 | 0.28 ± 0.16 | 0.38 ± 0.18 | 0.42 ± 0.17 | 0.46 ± 0.16 | 0.34 ± 0.16 |
| H08b-11w | 0.21 ± 0.11 | 0.33 ± 0.15 | 0.39 ± 0.16 | 0.43 ± 0.16 | 0.45 ± 0.16 | 0.36 ± 0.15 |
| H08b-15w | 0.21 ± 0.11 | 0.30 ± 0.12 | 0.35 ± 0.14 | 0.37 ± 0.15 | 0.36 ± 0.14 | 0.32 ± 0.13 |
| H16b-07w | 0.15 ± 0.11 | 0.23 ± 0.14 | 0.28 ± 0.16 | 0.28 ± 0.14 | 0.29 ± 0.15 | 0.25 ± 0.14 |
| H16b-11w | 0.20 ± 0.12 | 0.28 ± 0.15 | 0.31 ± 0.15 | 0.33 ± 0.15 | 0.37 ± 0.15 | 0.30 ± 0.14 |
| H16b-15w | 0.20 ± 0.11 | 0.26 ± 0.13 | 0.29 ± 0.13 | 0.31 ± 0.14 | 0.34 ± 0.14 | 0.28 ± 0.13 |
| H32b-07w | 0.08 ± 0.07 | 0.10 ± 0.08 | 0.14 ± 0.12 | 0.13 ± 0.12 | 0.12 ± 0.11 | 0.11 ± 0.10 |
| H32b-11w | 0.13 ± 0.09 | 0.18 ± 0.13 | 0.18 ± 0.13 | 0.18 ± 0.12 | 0.24 ± 0.12 | 0.18 ± 0.12 |
| H32b-15w | 0.14 ± 0.10 | 0.18 ± 0.13 | 0.19 ± 0.12 | 0.20 ± 0.10 | 0.26 ± 0.12 | 0.19 ± 0.11 |
| kNN-IP5n-cl1 | 0.33 ± 0.14 | 0.53 ± 0.17 | 0.66 ± 0.18 | 0.66 ± 0.20 | 0.64 ± 0.20 | 0.56 ± 0.18 |
| kNN-IP5n-cl2 | 0.34 ± 0.14 | 0.55 ± 0.17 | 0.71 ± 0.17 | 0.72 ± 0.19 | 0.68 ± 0.21 | 0.60 ± 0.18 |
| kNN-IP5n-cl3 | 0.34 ± 0.14 | 0.55 ± 0.17 | 0.72 ± 0.17 | 0.72 ± 0.18 | 0.67 ± 0.21 | 0.60 ± 0.18 |
| kNN-IP5n-cl4 | 0.34 ± 0.13 | 0.55 ± 0.17 | 0.71 ± 0.16 | 0.69 ± 0.16 | 0.60 ± 0.19 | 0.58 ± 0.16 |
| kNN-IP7n-cl1 | 0.34 ± 0.14 | 0.53 ± 0.17 | 0.63 ± 0.18 | 0.63 ± 0.20 | 0.61 ± 0.21 | 0.55 ± 0.18 |
| kNN-IP7n-cl2 | 0.34 ± 0.14 | 0.56 ± 0.18 | 0.72 ± 0.18 | 0.72 ± 0.19 | 0.66 ± 0.21 | 0.60 ± 0.18 |
| kNN-IP7n-cl3 | 0.35 ± 0.14 | 0.58 ± 0.18 | 0.73 ± 0.17 | 0.73 ± 0.18 | 0.68 ± 0.21 | 0.61 ± 0.18 |
| kNN-IP7n-cl4 | 0.35 ± 0.14 | 0.58 ± 0.18 | 0.74 ± 0.17 | 0.72 ± 0.17 | 0.64 ± 0.20 | 0.60 ± 0.17 |

**Table 6.1:** Performance of different appearance models on liver CT images for all resolutions $R_0$ (original resolution) to $R_4$ (four times down-sampled). Profile models are labeled as intensity (IP) or gradient profile (GP), followed by their length and an 'o' for original values or 'n' for normalized values. Histogram models are labeled by their number of bins ('b') and the width of the region they are collected in ('w'). For the clustered models, the clustering strategy is given as cl1 to cl4 – see the text for details. All results are given as mean and standard deviation.

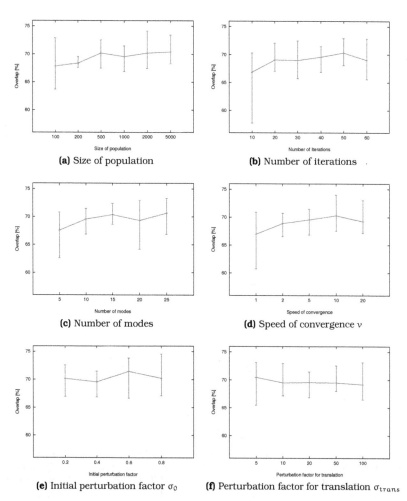

(a) Size of population       (b) Number of iterations

(c) Number of modes       (d) Speed of convergence $\nu$

(e) Initial perturbation factor $\sigma_0$       (f) Perturbation factor for translation $\sigma_{trans}$

**Figure 6.5:** Performance of the evolutionary algorithm for initialization of the liver model with different parameter sets. For each parameter value, the mean volumetric overlap is given, with error bars spanning the distance from lowest to highest overlap among the five test images.

| Resolution | Convergence criterion | $\gamma$ | $\Delta$ |
|---|---|---|---|
| 4 | $d_{max} < 4.0$ mm | - | - |
| 3 | $d_{max} < 2.0$ mm | - | - |
| 3 | $d_{max} < 0.3$ mm | 0.01 | 1 |
| 2 | $d_{max} < 0.4$ mm | 0.02 | 2 |
| 2 | $d_{max} < 1.0$ mm | 0.05 | 2 |
| 2 | $I = 50$ | 0.10 | 2 |
| 1 | $I = 50$ | 0.10 | 2 |

**Table 6.2:** Parameter values used in various phases of liver segmentation. A hyphen '-' for $\gamma$ signifies that the force equilibrium scheme was not used and the surface was restricted to the SSM. A hyphen for $\Delta$ means that the standard ASM optimization was used instead of the optimal surface search.

| Measure | Def | App-PW | No-OS | No-FD | App-Std [a] |
|---|---|---|---|---|---|
| VOE [%] | $8.3 \pm 3.5$ | $7.9 \pm 3.4$ | $9.7 \pm 5.3$ | $11.3 \pm 3.8$ | $34.7 \pm 14.1$ |
| RVD [%] | $2.7 \pm 4.7$ | $2.3 \pm 4.9$ | $1.1 \pm 7.2$ | $-0.4 \pm 3.8$ | $-31.6 \pm 14.9$ |
| ASD [mm] | $1.5 \pm 1.0$ | $1.5 \pm 1.0$ | $1.8 \pm 1.2$ | $2.0 \pm 1.2$ | $6.5 \pm 2.9$ |
| RMSSD [mm] | $3.5 \pm 2.5$ | $3.4 \pm 2.6$ | $4.1 \pm 3.0$ | $3.4 \pm 2.7$ | $10.4 \pm 4.1$ |
| MSD [mm] | $34.0 \pm 17.5$ | $32.9 \pm 17.7$ | $36.3 \pm 18.2$ | $30.4 \pm 19.6$ | $50.2 \pm 18.6$ |

[a]One segmentation attempt failed and was thus omitted from the statistics.

**Table 6.3:** Final segmentation results for the liver for various search strategies.

Following the obtained results, a final set of parameters was compiled to be used in the generation of the final initialization for all images. The chosen parameters were: 10 shape parameters, 1000 individuals in the population, 25 iterations, $\sigma_0 = 0.6$, $\sigma = 0.905$, $\nu = 10$, and $\sigma_{trans} = 10$. Utilizing these values, the evolutionary algorithm took approximately 5–6 minutes on a standard desktop PC to find a suitable initialization.

### Iterative search

While the parameters for the initialization of the model were still possible to evaluate systematically (at least when varying only one parameter at once), the enormous amount of possiblities of how to conduct multi-resolution iterative search made such a procedure impractical. Though it is usual to start at lower resolutions, the criteria for switching to the next-highest resolution can be chosen almost arbitrarily. In each resolution the amount of internal and external forces, the number of probes to take on each side of the deformable surface, the distance between these probes, and the maxi-

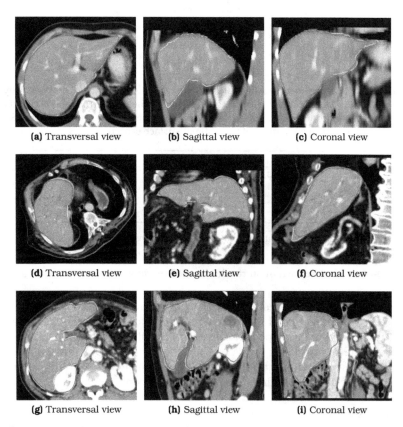

**(a)** Transversal view    **(b)** Sagittal view    **(c)** Coronal view

**(d)** Transversal view    **(e)** Sagittal view    **(f)** Coronal view

**(g)** Transversal view    **(h)** Sagittal view    **(i)** Coronal view

**Figure 6.6:** Selected slices of segmentation results on different licer CT images: the result of the presented search algorithm is displayed in red, the manually traced reference contour in green. Top row (a–c): image representing the $Q_{0.05}$ quantile of average surface distances – one of the best segmentations. Center row (d–f): image representing the median of average surface distances – an average result. Bottom row (g–i): image representing the $Q_{0.95}$ quantile of average surface distances – one of the failed segmentations.

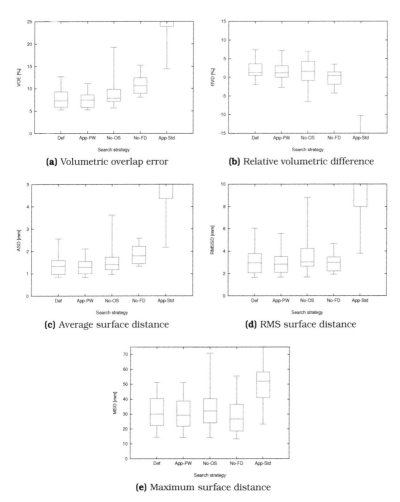

**(a)** Volumetric overlap error

**(b)** Relative volumetric difference

**(c)** Average surface distance

**(d)** RMS surface distance

**(e)** Maximum surface distance

**Figure 6.7:** Performance of different iterative search strategies for liver CT images. Box-plots show the median and the surrounding quartiles of the specific quality measure over all 45 images, with the whiskers indicating 5% and 95% quantiles. Results are shown for the developed default algorithm (Def), performance-weighted appearance models (App-PW), no optimal surface detection (No-OS), no free deformation (No-FD) and a standard Gaussian appearance model (App-Std).

mum allowed deviation $\Delta$ for the optimal surface detection, have an impact on the resulting segmentation. As a basis for the experiments conducted here, parameters determined empirically during an earlier study [100] were employed.

According to that study, parameters for the internal forces were set to $\alpha = 0.125$ and $\beta = 0.25$. The underlying shape model was restricted to $c = 10$ modes of variation, which explain approximately 90% of total variance encountered in the training data. The external forces were updated every $N_U = 10$ iterations. $K = 6$ probes were evaluated per side and landmark. The distance between two probes $d_P$ was set to 0.5 mm for the original resolution $R_0$. The parameters for the external forces were varied depending on the current phase of the search. In each phase, the deformable model was updated in its evolution according to Eq. 5.2 until a convergence criterion was met. Used input for these convergence criteria were maximum vertex movement $d_{max}$ after $N_U$ iterations and the number of iterations I for Eq. 5.2. The used values for liver segmentation are listed in Table 6.2. Per default, no weighting scheme for the fitting costs of the appearance model was used.

After convergence of the last phase, the resulting surface meshes were converted to binary image volumes the same size as the input data and stored for evaluation. Figure 6.6 displays the obtained segmentation results together with the manual reference contours for three different cases: a very accurate segmentation, a typical segmentation and a failed attempt.

To evaluate the impact of the different developments presented in this thesis, all images were also segmented with slightly varying strategies. The first modification was to employ the weighting of fitting costs according to the calculated performance indices. Subsequently, the optimal surface detection was not included and the minimum-fitting-costs rule was used to determine landmark candidate positions in each iteration. Another variant was to leave out the free deformation and use hard shape constraints for all phases. To allow more flexibility, all available modes of variation were used in this variant. Finally, instead of using the clustered non-linear appearance model, a conventional Gaussian model was utilized for segmentation. The corresponding normalized intensity profile of length 7 was selected for this purpose. A quantitative comparison between all variants is given in Fig. 6.7, which shows box-plots for all measures of segmentation accuracy presented in Sec. 5.5. Exact numbers of mean and standard deviation are given in Table 6.3. The best result was reached by the search method using

free deformation, optimal surface detection and weighted costs for the non-linear appearance models. For this variant, the average surface distance was 1.5 mm and the overlap error 7.9%. On a standard desktop PC, the search took less than 3 minutes per image.

### 6.1.5 Performance index verification

As concluding experiment for the liver, it was evaluated in how far the performance indices calculated for different appearance models in Sec. 6.1.3 correlated to real-world results. Using search parameters determined in the previous section, the standard deformable search algorithm was run on five random images for all appearance models. The resulting segmentations were assessed using volumetric overlap measure and correlated with a weighted average of the previously calculated performance indices $\xi$.

Correct or incorrect boundary detection in the rougher resolution levels has a greater impact on the final segmentation result than in the finer resolution levels. For this reason, the performance index of a rougher resolution level was weighted higher than the indices of lower levels. As image resolution is always halved with each down-sampling step, a factor of 2 was chosen for weighting. Given the search scheme for the liver in Table 6.2, this results in the following average performance index:

$$\bar{\xi} = \frac{1}{30} \left( 2\xi(R_1) + 4\xi(R_2) + 8\xi(R_3) + 16\xi(R_4) \right) \tag{6.1}$$

Figure 6.8 shows the relation between this weighted performance index and the obtained segmentation result. The Pearson correlation coefficient between the two variables is $r = 0.66$. When ignoring the three outlier samples at the bottom (the local histograms with 32 bins which failed completely), the correlation coefficient increases to $r = 0.73$.

## 6.2 Evaluation on the lung (MRI)

The medical motivation for segmenting lung lobes from MRI images originates from a study that is currently conducted at the radiology department of the German Cancer Research Center [196]. In this study, it is examined in how far MRI can be used to amend the currently employed technique of spirometry to assess pulmonary function. In spirometry, the volume of air a patient can inhale and exhale in one breath is measured – this corresponds to the volume of both lung lobes. In case of diseases where only

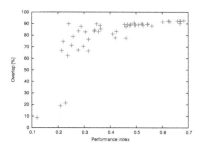

**Figure 6.8:** Correlation between the average performance index $\bar{\xi}$ and the quality of the corresponding segmentation for the liver CT data. To estimate the quality of segmentation, five images were segmented for each appearance model, the volumetric overlaps with the references were calculated and averaged.

one lung lobe is affected locally (e.g. by a tumor), this technique is not accurate enough to detect the difference. Therefore, the aim is to detect such local problems more reliably on a sequence of 3D images over the breathing cycle. A key requisite for this new method however is a robust method for lung segmentation.

### 6.2.1 Data material

To achieve an acquisition time that is fast enough to capture moving lungs without blur, spatial resolution must be decreased drastically. Images used for this experiment were acquired using a special FLASH sequence that resulted in 96x128x52 voxels per volume with a voxel spacing of 3.75x3.75x 3.8 mm. Nine patients were examined, and for each one, 20 image volumes were acquired over the breathing cycle. In each volume, both lung lobes were segmented semi-automatically in slice-by-slice fashion by a medical expert. For simplicity, the left lobe was chosen as object of interest for this experiment – it could also have been the right one, and obviously both models must be built and used to serve a clinical purpose. Due to topology problems with some of the images, 166 volumes were finally selected for inclusion in the statistical model.

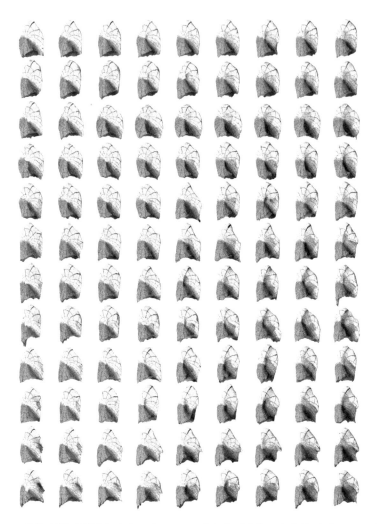

**Figure 6.9:** 108 of 166 training shapes used to build the statistical shape model of the left lung lobe. Detected point-correspondences are visualized using a color-coded coordinate grid.

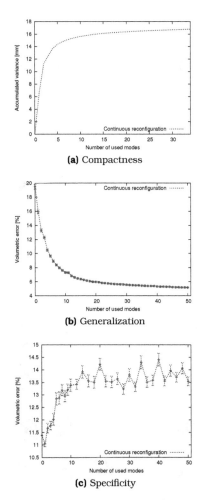

**(a)** Compactness

**(b)** Generalization

**(c)** Specificity

**Figure 6.10:** Quantitative evaluation of the lung model.

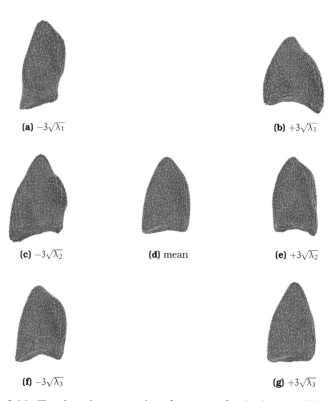

**(a)** $-3\sqrt{\lambda_1}$          **(b)** $+3\sqrt{\lambda_1}$

**(c)** $-3\sqrt{\lambda_2}$      **(d)** mean      **(e)** $+3\sqrt{\lambda_2}$

**(f)** $-3\sqrt{\lambda_3}$          **(g)** $+3\sqrt{\lambda_3}$

**Figure 6.11:** The three largest modes of variation for the lung model. For each mode, the shapes at a distance of three standard deviations from the mean are displayed.

### 6.2.2 Shape model construction

Surfaces extracted from the 166 training volumes consisted of approximately 1000 vertices, so an equal number of landmarks was utilized for the shape model. Since no fixed landmark template with 1000 points on the sphere was available, point correspondences were determined only with the continuous landmark reconfiguration from Sec. 3.4. As in case of the liver, reconfiguration was employed every 10 iterations. The entire process took approximately 50 hours on a standard desktop PC.

Resulting correspondences are displayed in Fig. 6.9, which overlays a common coordinate-grid to all shapes. Compactness, generalization and specificity of the obtained model are displayed in Fig. 6.10. For better understanding of the encountered variation, the three largest eigenmodes are shown in Fig. 6.11.

### 6.2.3 Appearance models

The general process of evaluating different appearance models was very similar to the liver experiment. First, 20 images were randomly selected and excluded from all training. Using the remaining 146 images, the following appearance models were built: 8 Gaussian intensity profile models (normalized and unnormalized versions, each with lengths of 3, 5, 7 and 9 samples), 8 Gaussian gradient profile models, 8 non-linear intensity profile models and 8 non-linear gradient profile models (all using the same variations of length and normalization). Due to the lower resolution of the training images, the profile spacing was set to 3.75 mm for this application. In addition to the 32 profile models, 9 histogram models were constructed with varying number of bins and varying size of the sample region. As for the liver, performance evaluation followed the process described in Sec. 4.3. Detailed results are listed in Table 6.4, Fig. 6.12 shows the corresponding box-plots as an overview.

With an average performance index of 0.64, the 7 samples long normalized gradient profile non-linear model reached the best result and was chosen for clustering. Using varying parameters for the mean-shift algorithm, four clustered models were created. The first model featured 227 clusters, the second 52, the third 8 and the forth combined all data into one single boundary model. Following the good results obtained for the liver model, the next largest profile model (i.e. 9 samples long) of the same type also underwent the clustering process, resulting in 224, 54, 8 and one cluster.

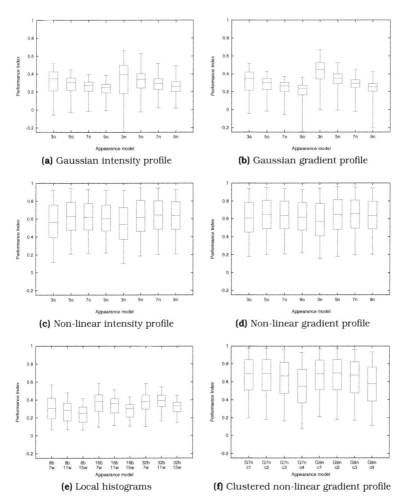

**Figure 6.12:** Performance of different appearance models on the lung MRI images. Box-plots show median and surrounding quartiles of calculated performance index over all landmarks and all resolutions. Whiskers indicate the 5% and 95% quantiles. Profile models are labeled by their length, followed by an 'o' for original values or 'n' for normalized values. The histogram models are labeled by their number of bins ('b') and the width of the region they are collected in ('w'). For the clustered models, the clustering strategy is given as c1 to c4 – see the text for details.

The 8 new appearance models were also evaluated and their performance added to Table 6.4 and Fig. 6.12.

### 6.2.4 Segmentation results

Cross-validation was employed with 8 sets of images to evaluate the final performance of segmentation with the lung model. In each set, 20 images were left out. All correspondences are based on the initial optimization with continuous landmark reconfiguration. For each set, a normalized gradient profile appearance model of length 7 was built, in its clustered non-linear variant (NGP7-kNN-cl1 in Table. 6.4).

#### Initialization

Due to the lower number of landmarks (in comparison to the liver model), the minimum geodesic radius in which a landmark must exist was set to $r = 1$ for the model decimation step. This setting resulted in 193 landmarks for the reduced model. The global search was conducted in the twice down-sampled images ($R_2$), as further down-sampling did not seem to be useful with the low resolution of input image data (only 52 voxels on the shortest side).

To determine a suitable set of parameters for the genetic algorithm, the same series of tests as for the liver data was conducted. Each parameter set was tested on 10 randomly selected images. The results of these experiments are summarized in Fig. 6.13. As most of the resulting graphs are relatively stable to parameter changes, the compilation of the final parameter set was also influenced by considerations regarding the speed of computation (smaller populations and fewer iterations being the fastest). The following values were chosen for the subsequent experiments: 15 shape parameters, 1000 individuals in the population, 20 iterations, $\sigma_0 = 0.4$, $\sigma = 0.9$, $v = 5$, and $\sigma_{trans} = 10$. This configuration resulted in an average runtime of less than 2 minutes per image on a standard desktop PC.

#### Iterative search

As the shape of the left lung lobe does not vary as much as the liver, convergence criteria for different phases of the iterative search should not be too critical: Less variation means that the distance of the model to the true contour is generally smaller, and if the model does not converge completely

| App-Model | $R_0$ | $R_1$ | $R_2$ | $R_3$ | $R_4$ | Average |
|---|---|---|---|---|---|---|
| Gauss-IP3o | $0.28 \pm 0.12$ | $0.37 \pm 0.10$ | $0.38 \pm 0.11$ | $0.28 \pm 0.16$ | $0.23 \pm 0.20$ | $0.31 \pm 0.14$ |
| Gauss-IP5o | $0.23 \pm 0.10$ | $0.30 \pm 0.08$ | $0.32 \pm 0.08$ | $0.27 \pm 0.10$ | $0.26 \pm 0.19$ | $0.28 \pm 0.12$ |
| Gauss-IP7o | $0.20 \pm 0.08$ | $0.26 \pm 0.07$ | $0.28 \pm 0.06$ | $0.26 \pm 0.07$ | $0.23 \pm 0.16$ | $0.25 \pm 0.10$ |
| Gauss-IP9o | $0.17 \pm 0.07$ | $0.23 \pm 0.06$ | $0.26 \pm 0.05$ | $0.25 \pm 0.06$ | $0.23 \pm 0.16$ | $0.23 \pm 0.09$ |
| Gauss-IP3n | $0.25 \pm 0.15$ | $0.38 \pm 0.16$ | $0.43 \pm 0.17$ | $0.29 \pm 0.27$ | $0.27 \pm 0.33$ | $0.32 \pm 0.23$ |
| Gauss-IP5n | $0.24 \pm 0.10$ | $0.32 \pm 0.10$ | $0.36 \pm 0.11$ | $0.31 \pm 0.12$ | $0.38 \pm 0.25$ | $0.32 \pm 0.15$ |
| Gauss-IP7n | $0.21 \pm 0.08$ | $0.28 \pm 0.07$ | $0.31 \pm 0.08$ | $0.29 \pm 0.08$ | $0.33 \pm 0.20$ | $0.28 \pm 0.11$ |
| Gauss-IP9n | $0.18 \pm 0.07$ | $0.24 \pm 0.06$ | $0.27 \pm 0.07$ | $0.27 \pm 0.07$ | $0.31 \pm 0.19$ | $0.25 \pm 0.11$ |
| Gauss-GP3o | $0.26 \pm 0.13$ | $0.34 \pm 0.13$ | $0.36 \pm 0.13$ | $0.28 \pm 0.14$ | $0.31 \pm 0.18$ | $0.31 \pm 0.14$ |
| Gauss-GP5o | $0.22 \pm 0.10$ | $0.30 \pm 0.07$ | $0.32 \pm 0.07$ | $0.29 \pm 0.09$ | $0.24 \pm 0.19$ | $0.27 \pm 0.11$ |
| Gauss-GP7o | $0.19 \pm 0.08$ | $0.25 \pm 0.06$ | $0.28 \pm 0.06$ | $0.26 \pm 0.06$ | $0.21 \pm 0.21$ | $0.24 \pm 0.11$ |
| Gauss-GP9o | $0.16 \pm 0.07$ | $0.22 \pm 0.06$ | $0.26 \pm 0.05$ | $0.23 \pm 0.06$ | $0.13 \pm 0.28$ | $0.20 \pm 0.13$ |
| Gauss-GP3n | $0.38 \pm 0.12$ | $0.45 \pm 0.12$ | $0.47 \pm 0.12$ | $0.38 \pm 0.15$ | $0.43 \pm 0.23$ | $0.42 \pm 0.16$ |
| Gauss-GP5n | $0.29 \pm 0.08$ | $0.35 \pm 0.07$ | $0.37 \pm 0.07$ | $0.34 \pm 0.10$ | $0.31 \pm 0.22$ | $0.33 \pm 0.12$ |
| Gauss-GP7n | $0.24 \pm 0.07$ | $0.29 \pm 0.06$ | $0.31 \pm 0.06$ | $0.30 \pm 0.07$ | $0.24 \pm 0.23$ | $0.28 \pm 0.12$ |
| Gauss-GP9n | $0.20 \pm 0.06$ | $0.25 \pm 0.05$ | $0.28 \pm 0.06$ | $0.26 \pm 0.05$ | $0.16 \pm 0.28$ | $0.23 \pm 0.14$ |
| kNN-IP3o | $0.38 \pm 0.14$ | $0.60 \pm 0.16$ | $0.73 \pm 0.16$ | $0.60 \pm 0.23$ | $0.49 \pm 0.26$ | $0.56 \pm 0.20$ |
| kNN-IP5o | $0.40 \pm 0.14$ | $0.62 \pm 0.17$ | $0.75 \pm 0.15$ | $0.69 \pm 0.16$ | $0.63 \pm 0.20$ | $0.62 \pm 0.17$ |
| kNN-IP7o | $0.40 \pm 0.13$ | $0.61 \pm 0.16$ | $0.73 \pm 0.15$ | $0.69 \pm 0.15$ | $0.64 \pm 0.20$ | $0.61 \pm 0.16$ |
| kNN-IP9o | $0.40 \pm 0.13$ | $0.59 \pm 0.15$ | $0.70 \pm 0.15$ | $0.67 \pm 0.15$ | $0.65 \pm 0.20$ | $0.60 \pm 0.16$ |
| kNN-IP3n | $0.34 \pm 0.13$ | $0.57 \pm 0.18$ | $0.70 \pm 0.16$ | $0.60 \pm 0.21$ | $0.48 \pm 0.24$ | $0.54 \pm 0.19$ |
| kNN-IP5n | $0.38 \pm 0.14$ | $0.62 \pm 0.19$ | $0.75 \pm 0.15$ | $0.72 \pm 0.17$ | $0.62 \pm 0.21$ | $0.62 \pm 0.17$ |
| kNN-IP7n | $0.39 \pm 0.14$ | $0.63 \pm 0.17$ | $0.75 \pm 0.14$ | $0.73 \pm 0.15$ | $0.64 \pm 0.20$ | $0.63 \pm 0.16$ |
| kNN-IP9n | $0.40 \pm 0.14$ | $0.62 \pm 0.16$ | $0.72 \pm 0.14$ | $0.72 \pm 0.15$ | $0.66 \pm 0.20$ | $0.62 \pm 0.16$ |
| kNN-GP3o | $0.39 \pm 0.14$ | $0.61 \pm 0.18$ | $0.75 \pm 0.16$ | $0.66 \pm 0.17$ | $0.62 \pm 0.21$ | $0.60 \pm 0.17$ |
| kNN-GP5o | $0.40 \pm 0.14$ | $0.64 \pm 0.17$ | $0.78 \pm 0.14$ | $0.71 \pm 0.16$ | $0.64 \pm 0.20$ | $0.63 \pm 0.17$ |
| kNN-GP7o | $0.41 \pm 0.14$ | $0.62 \pm 0.17$ | $0.76 \pm 0.14$ | $0.70 \pm 0.16$ | $0.66 \pm 0.20$ | $0.63 \pm 0.16$ |
| kNN-GP9o | $0.40 \pm 0.14$ | $0.61 \pm 0.16$ | $0.74 \pm 0.15$ | $0.68 \pm 0.16$ | $0.66 \pm 0.20$ | $0.62 \pm 0.16$ |
| kNN-GP3n | $0.35 \pm 0.14$ | $0.58 \pm 0.19$ | $0.73 \pm 0.15$ | $0.65 \pm 0.19$ | $0.57 \pm 0.23$ | $0.58 \pm 0.18$ |
| kNN-GP5n | $0.39 \pm 0.14$ | $0.64 \pm 0.18$ | $0.78 \pm 0.14$ | $0.73 \pm 0.16$ | $0.63 \pm 0.21$ | $0.63 \pm 0.17$ |
| kNN-GP7n | $0.40 \pm 0.14$ | $0.64 \pm 0.17$ | $0.77 \pm 0.14$ | $0.73 \pm 0.15$ | $0.65 \pm 0.21$ | $0.64 \pm 0.16$ |
| kNN-GP9n | $0.40 \pm 0.14$ | $0.63 \pm 0.16$ | $0.75 \pm 0.14$ | $0.71 \pm 0.15$ | $0.65 \pm 0.21$ | $0.63 \pm 0.16$ |
| H08b-07w | $0.17 \pm 0.11$ | $0.24 \pm 0.12$ | $0.34 \pm 0.11$ | $0.32 \pm 0.08$ | $0.46 \pm 0.08$ | $0.31 \pm 0.10$ |
| H08b-11w | $0.16 \pm 0.10$ | $0.22 \pm 0.10$ | $0.25 \pm 0.08$ | $0.34 \pm 0.09$ | $0.39 \pm 0.05$ | $0.27 \pm 0.08$ |
| H08b-15w | $0.14 \pm 0.07$ | $0.18 \pm 0.08$ | $0.22 \pm 0.06$ | $0.31 \pm 0.06$ | $0.35 \pm 0.06$ | $0.24 \pm 0.07$ |
| H16b-07w | $0.24 \pm 0.13$ | $0.34 \pm 0.13$ | $0.41 \pm 0.11$ | $0.39 \pm 0.07$ | $0.45 \pm 0.08$ | $0.37 \pm 0.11$ |
| H16b-11w | $0.25 \pm 0.12$ | $0.33 \pm 0.11$ | $0.33 \pm 0.09$ | $0.38 \pm 0.08$ | $0.40 \pm 0.05$ | $0.34 \pm 0.09$ |
| H16b-15w | $0.21 \pm 0.09$ | $0.25 \pm 0.09$ | $0.27 \pm 0.07$ | $0.32 \pm 0.06$ | $0.36 \pm 0.05$ | $0.28 \pm 0.07$ |
| H32b-07w | $0.26 \pm 0.13$ | $0.36 \pm 0.12$ | $0.43 \pm 0.11$ | $0.38 \pm 0.07$ | $0.42 \pm 0.09$ | $0.37 \pm 0.11$ |
| H32b-11w | $0.31 \pm 0.12$ | $0.40 \pm 0.11$ | $0.40 \pm 0.09$ | $0.40 \pm 0.08$ | $0.41 \pm 0.06$ | $0.38 \pm 0.09$ |
| H32b-15w | $0.27 \pm 0.09$ | $0.32 \pm 0.09$ | $0.30 \pm 0.07$ | $0.34 \pm 0.06$ | $0.36 \pm 0.05$ | $0.32 \pm 0.07$ |
| kNN-GP7n-cl1 | $0.40 \pm 0.14$ | $0.66 \pm 0.18$ | $0.81 \pm 0.14$ | $0.78 \pm 0.15$ | $0.67 \pm 0.21$ | $0.66 \pm 0.17$ |
| kNN-GP7n-cl2 | $0.39 \pm 0.14$ | $0.66 \pm 0.18$ | $0.81 \pm 0.14$ | $0.77 \pm 0.16$ | $0.65 \pm 0.22$ | $0.66 \pm 0.17$ |
| kNN-GP7n-cl3 | $0.37 \pm 0.14$ | $0.64 \pm 0.18$ | $0.79 \pm 0.13$ | $0.74 \pm 0.17$ | $0.62 \pm 0.22$ | $0.63 \pm 0.17$ |
| kNN-GP7n-cl4 | $0.32 \pm 0.14$ | $0.57 \pm 0.19$ | $0.75 \pm 0.13$ | $0.68 \pm 0.18$ | $0.40 \pm 0.20$ | $0.54 \pm 0.17$ |
| kNN-GP9n-cl1 | $0.40 \pm 0.14$ | $0.66 \pm 0.17$ | $0.80 \pm 0.13$ | $0.77 \pm 0.15$ | $0.67 \pm 0.21$ | $0.66 \pm 0.16$ |
| kNN-GP9n-cl2 | $0.40 \pm 0.14$ | $0.67 \pm 0.18$ | $0.81 \pm 0.13$ | $0.78 \pm 0.15$ | $0.66 \pm 0.23$ | $0.66 \pm 0.17$ |
| kNN-GP9n-cl3 | $0.38 \pm 0.14$ | $0.63 \pm 0.18$ | $0.79 \pm 0.13$ | $0.76 \pm 0.16$ | $0.63 \pm 0.22$ | $0.64 \pm 0.17$ |
| kNN-GP9n-cl4 | $0.33 \pm 0.14$ | $0.58 \pm 0.19$ | $0.77 \pm 0.14$ | $0.72 \pm 0.17$ | $0.42 \pm 0.19$ | $0.56 \pm 0.17$ |

**Table 6.4:** Performance of different appearance models on lung MRI images for all resolutions $R_0$ (original resolution) to $R_4$ (four times down-sampled). Profile models are labeled as intensity (IP) or gradient profile (GP), followed by their length and an 'o' for original values or 'n' for normalized values. Histogram models are labeled by their number of bins ('b') and the width of the region they are collected in ('w'). For the clustered models, the clustering strategy is given as cl1 to cl4 – see the text for details. All results are given as mean and standard deviation.

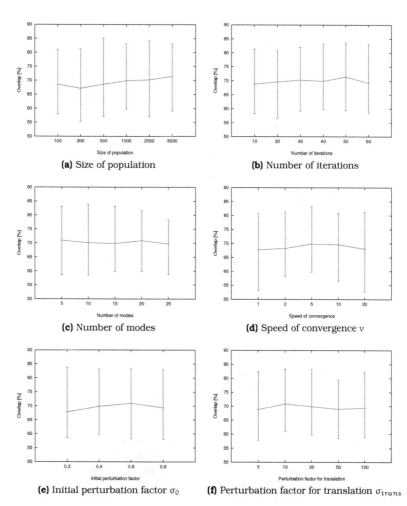

**Figure 6.13:** Performance of the evolutionary algorithm for initialization of the lung model with different parameter sets. For each parameter value, the mean volumetric overlap is given, with error bars spanning the distance from lowest to highest overlap among the ten test images.

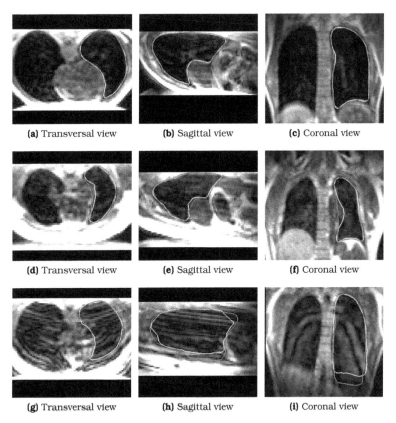

**(a)** Transversal view  **(b)** Sagittal view  **(c)** Coronal view

**(d)** Transversal view  **(e)** Sagittal view  **(f)** Coronal view

**(g)** Transversal view  **(h)** Sagittal view  **(i)** Coronal view

**Figure 6.14:** Selected slices of segmentation results on different lung MRI images: the result of the presented search algorithm is displayed in red, the manually traced reference contour in green. Top row (a–c): image representing the $Q_{0.05}$ quantile of average surface distances – one of the best segmentations. Center row (d–f): image representing the median of average surface distances – an average result. Bottom row (g–i): image representing the $Q_{0.95}$ quantile of average surface distances – one of the failed segmentations.

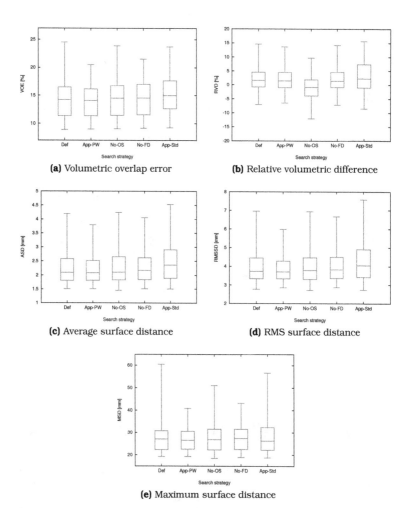

**(a)** Volumetric overlap error

**(b)** Relative volumetric difference

**(c)** Average surface distance

**(d)** RMS surface distance

**(e)** Maximum surface distance

**Figure 6.15:** Performance of different iterative search strategies for lung MRI images. Box-plots show the median and the surrounding quartiles of the specific quality measure over all 45 images, with the whiskers indicating 5% and 95% quantiles. Results are shown for the developed default algorithm (Def), performance-weighted appearance models (App-PW), no optimal surface detection (No-OS), no free deformation (No-FD) and a standard Gaussian appearance model (App-Std).

| Resolution | Convergence criterion | $\gamma$ | $\Delta$ |
|---|---|---|---|
| 2 | $d_{max} < 1.0$ mm | - | 1 |
| 1 | $d_{max} < 0.75$ mm | - | 1 |
| 1 | $I = 100$ | 0.05 | 1 |
| 0 | $I = 100$ | 0.10 | 2 |

**Table 6.5:** Parameter values used in various phases of lung segmentation. A hyphen '-' for $\gamma$ signifies that the force equilibrium scheme was not used and the surface was restricted to the SSM.

| Measure | Def | App-PW | No-OS | No-FD | App-Std |
|---|---|---|---|---|---|
| VOE [%] | $15.1 \pm 6.4$ | $14.3 \pm 4.1$ | $15.1 \pm 5.2$ | $14.9 \pm 4.7$ | $15.8 \pm 5.3$ |
| RVD [%] | $2.3 \pm 10.9$ | $2.3 \pm 7.0$ | $-1.1 \pm 7.6$ | $2.3 \pm 7.5$ | $3.1 \pm 8.2$ |
| ASD [mm] | $2.6 \pm 1.8$ | $2.3 \pm 1.0$ | $2.5 \pm 1.5$ | $2.4 \pm 1.2$ | $2.6 \pm 1.4$ |
| RMSSD [mm] | $4.7 \pm 3.6$ | $4.2 \pm 2.0$ | $4.4 \pm 3.0$ | $4.3 \pm 2.1$ | $4.6 \pm 2.5$ |
| MSD [mm] | $30.2 \pm 15.6$ | $28.2 \pm 9.9$ | $29.6 \pm 13.1$ | $28.9 \pm 9.8$ | $29.7 \pm 13.1$ |

**Table 6.6:** Final segmentation results for the left lung lobe for various search strategies.

in one level of resolution, the errors can often still be corrected at the following level. As the initialization was previously conducted in resolution $R_2$, some refinement was conducted before switching to $R_1$. Free deformation started in the third phase (still in $R_1$), and final adjustments were made in the original resolution $R_0$. Table 6.5 gives an overview of the used settings. As in the initialization, the shape model was restricted to 15 modes of variation during the iterative search, which corresponds to 90% of total variance encountered in the training set. Internal forces were set to the identical values as for the liver, where $\alpha = 0.125$ and $\beta = 0.25$. External forces were updated every 10 iterations. $K = 6$ probes were taken at each side of the surface during search, due to the low resolution of the images the distance between two probes was set to $d_p = 1.5$ mm. No weighting scheme for the appearance models was used in the default configuration.

Qualitative results of segmentation are displayed in Fig. 6.14, which shows the obtained contours for three different cases. Again, a very accurate segmentation, a typical case and a failed attempt were chosen. Quantitative results for the default search strategy and the four variants appearance performance weighting, no optimal surface detection, no free deformation, and standard appearance model (normalized gradient profile of length 7) are given in Fig. 6.15. The corresponding numbers for mean and standard deviation are listed in Table 6.6. As in case of the liver, the most

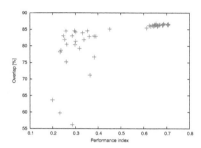

**Figure 6.16:** Correlation between the average performance index $\bar{\xi}$ and the quality the corresponding segmentation for the lung MRI data. To estimate the quality of segmentation, five images were segmented for each appearance model, the volumetric overlaps with the references were calculated and averaged.

accurate results were obtained with free deformation, optimal surface detection and weighting of appearance costs: Using this configuration, the average surface distance was 2.3 mm and the volumetric error 14.3%. On a standard PC, the iterative search process took approximately 20 seconds per image.

### 6.2.5 Performance index verification

As for the liver, experiments on the lung images were cóncluded with verifying the theoretical performance indices for the appearance models. The weighted average $\bar{\xi}$ for each model was calculated according to the search strategy for the lung (as listed in Table 6.5), which resulted in:

$$\bar{\xi} = \frac{1}{7}\left(\xi(R_0) + 2\xi(R_1) + 4\xi(R_2)\right) \tag{6.2}$$

Figure 6.8 shows the relation between this weighted performance index and the obtained segmentation result. The Pearson correlation coefficient between the two variables is $r = 0.63$. As before, there are three outlier samples with very low performance (the local histogram models with 8 bins), which when omitted from the calculation, let the correlation coefficient increase to $r = 0.73$.

## 6.3 Evaluation on the prostate (US)

One of the navigation projects in the German Cancer Research Center is concerned with image-guided prostate surgery [8]. In this project, 3D ultrasound images acquired during surgery must be matched to preoperative CT data. As registering US to CT is a challenging problem, an alternative solution is to segment the ultrasound data and match the extracted shape instead. A model-based segmentation has the advantage that once the object of interest is found, it can be tracked over time without requiring too much processing power.

### 6.3.1 Data material

Images used in this experiment are 35 trans-rectal ultrasound volumes with a resolution varying between 430x280x200 voxels and 480x430x250 voxels. Voxel spacing varies from 0.15 to 0.2 mm in-plane and from 0.2 to 0.25 mm between consecutive slices. Although the physical resolution is very good, US is one of the noisier modalities in medical imaging, and as such, the data is commonly filtered before processing. For this experiment, a 7x7x7 median filter was employed to smooth all images beforehand. Reference segmentations of the prostate were created by a trained medical student using manually controlled deformable simplex meshes [15]. As can be seen in Fig. 6.17, the prostate has a relatively simple shape without protruding features.

### 6.3.2 Shape model construction

As the meshes defining the prostate segmentations were quite smooth, 642 landmarks (corresponding to 3 subdivision levels on an icosahedron) were deemed sufficient for an accurate representation of the shape. To evaluate the effects of landmark reconfiguration on simpler shapes, three different models were built (as for the liver): one using the standard gradient optimization, one a single reconfiguration step after convergence and one using continuous reconfiguration every 10 iterations. On a standard desktop PC, the entire correspondence optimization took approximately 0.5 hours without and 1.5 hours including continuous reconfiguration.

All three models were evaluated using compactness, generalization and specificity. The results are displayed in Fig. 6.18. As landmark reconfiguration did not bring any advantages in this case, the standard model was

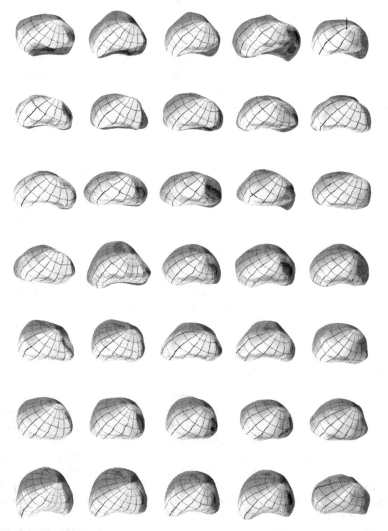

**Figure 6.17:** All 35 training shapes for the prostate model. Detected point correspondences are visualized using a color-coded coordinate grid.

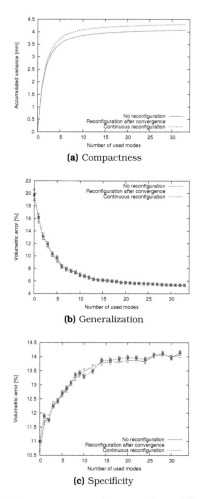

**(a)** Compactness

**(b)** Generalization

**(c)** Specificity

**Figure 6.18:** Quantitative comparison between three different optimization approaches for the prostate model.

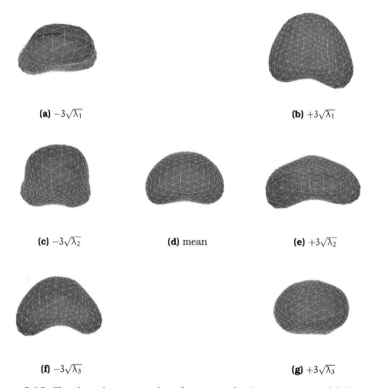

**(a)** $-3\sqrt{\lambda_1}$        **(b)** $+3\sqrt{\lambda_1}$

**(c)** $-3\sqrt{\lambda_2}$     **(d)** mean     **(e)** $+3\sqrt{\lambda_2}$

**(f)** $-3\sqrt{\lambda_3}$        **(g)** $+3\sqrt{\lambda_3}$

**Figure 6.19:** The three largest modes of variation for the prostate model. For each mode, the shapes three standard deviations away from the mean are displayed.

chosen as the basis for the following steps. Its largest modes of variation are shown in Fig. 6.19. Additionally, detected correspondences can also be inspected by the color-coded coordinate grid in Fig. 6.17.

### 6.3.3 Appearance Models

The identical procedure as for the other two applications was used to evaluate appearance models. Tests were run on 5 random images excluded from training. Again, 32 profiles models (8 Gaussian intensity, 8 Gaussian gradient, 8 non-linear intensity and 8 non-linear gradient) were built for the prostate. Following the guideline of adjusting the profile spacing according to the image resolution, a distance of 0.25 mm between two neighboring profile samples was chosen for the original resolution $R_0$. As the actual image content was too noisy, a fourth variant of the local histogram model with a 19x19x19 sized region was added to the other three sizes (7, 11 and 15 cube voxels), resulting in 12 different histogram models. Evaluating these models with the performance index from Sec. 4.3 led to the results presented in Fig. 6.20 and in Table 6.7.

Best results were obtained with 7 and 9 samples long gradient profile models, normalized and using the non-linear kNN classifier. Both models underwent the mean-shift clustering process with varying parameters for kernel size and minimum cluster size. For the 7 samples long profile, this resulted in 144, 35, 7 and 1 clusters, the 9 samples long profile was combined in a very similar way to 145, 35, 6, and 1 clusters, depending on the used parameters. Results for these 8 additional models are also available in the above mentioned figure and table. Overall, the best performance of 0.26 was reached with the 9 samples long profile clustered with strategy 2 (i.e. 35 resulting clusters).

### 6.3.4 Segmentation results

From the 35 prostate images, 7 sets were created for cross-validation, and in each set 5 (different) images were omitted from training. For each set, a shape model was built using the correspondences from the initial optimization without landmark reconfiguration. Subsequently, the corresponding appearance models were constructed, using the 9 samples long clustered non-linear normalized gradient profile type which performed best in the previous section.

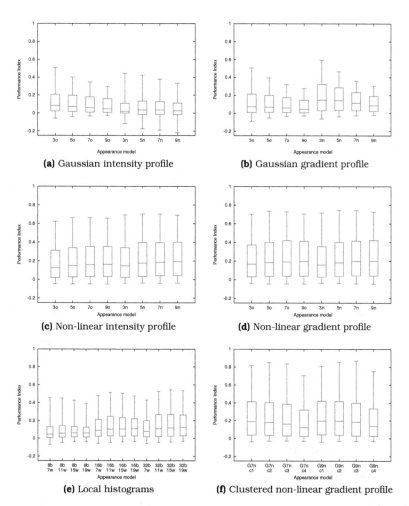

**Figure 6.20:** Performance of different appearance models on the prostate US images. Box-plots show median and surrounding quartiles of calculated performance index over all landmarks and all resolutions. Whiskers indicate the 5% and 95% quantiles. Profile models are labeled by their length, followed by an 'o' for original values or 'n' for normalized values. The histogram models are labeled by their number of bins ('b') and the width of the region they are collected in ('w'). For the clustered models, the clustering strategy is given as c1 to c4 – see the text for details.

| App-Model | $R_0$ | $R_1$ | $R_2$ | $R_3$ | $R_4$ | Average |
|---|---|---|---|---|---|---|
| Gauss-IP3o | $0.02 \pm 0.04$ | $0.05 \pm 0.07$ | $0.11 \pm 0.10$ | $0.18 \pm 0.14$ | $0.30 \pm 0.16$ | $0.13 \pm 0.11$ |
| Gauss-IP5o | $0.02 \pm 0.03$ | $0.04 \pm 0.06$ | $0.08 \pm 0.08$ | $0.18 \pm 0.12$ | $0.26 \pm 0.13$ | $0.11 \pm 0.09$ |
| Gauss-IP7o | $0.01 \pm 0.02$ | $0.03 \pm 0.05$ | $0.08 \pm 0.08$ | $0.15 \pm 0.10$ | $0.23 \pm 0.10$ | $0.10 \pm 0.08$ |
| Gauss-IP9o | $0.00 \pm 0.02$ | $0.03 \pm 0.04$ | $0.07 \pm 0.07$ | $0.13 \pm 0.09$ | $0.19 \pm 0.09$ | $0.09 \pm 0.07$ |
| Gauss-IP3n | $0.00 \pm 0.05$ | $0.02 \pm 0.07$ | $0.06 \pm 0.11$ | $0.09 \pm 0.15$ | $0.16 \pm 0.19$ | $0.07 \pm 0.13$ |
| Gauss-IP5n | $0.01 \pm 0.05$ | $0.03 \pm 0.08$ | $0.06 \pm 0.13$ | $0.10 \pm 0.17$ | $0.13 \pm 0.20$ | $0.06 \pm 0.14$ |
| Gauss-IP7n | $0.01 \pm 0.05$ | $0.02 \pm 0.08$ | $0.06 \pm 0.12$ | $0.09 \pm 0.15$ | $0.12 \pm 0.20$ | $0.06 \pm 0.13$ |
| Gauss-IP9n | $0.00 \pm 0.04$ | $0.03 \pm 0.08$ | $0.05 \pm 0.11$ | $0.06 \pm 0.15$ | $0.10 \pm 0.19$ | $0.05 \pm 0.12$ |
| Gauss-GP3o | $0.02 \pm 0.04$ | $0.04 \pm 0.07$ | $0.10 \pm 0.10$ | $0.20 \pm 0.16$ | $0.27 \pm 0.20$ | $0.12 \pm 0.13$ |
| Gauss-GP5o | $0.01 \pm 0.03$ | $0.03 \pm 0.06$ | $0.09 \pm 0.09$ | $0.18 \pm 0.13$ | $0.24 \pm 0.12$ | $0.11 \pm 0.09$ |
| Gauss-GP7o | $0.01 \pm 0.02$ | $0.03 \pm 0.05$ | $0.08 \pm 0.07$ | $0.15 \pm 0.10$ | $0.21 \pm 0.09$ | $0.09 \pm 0.07$ |
| Gauss-GP9o | $0.00 \pm 0.02$ | $0.03 \pm 0.04$ | $0.06 \pm 0.06$ | $0.12 \pm 0.08$ | $0.18 \pm 0.08$ | $0.08 \pm 0.06$ |
| Gauss-GP3n | $0.03 \pm 0.07$ | $0.10 \pm 0.12$ | $0.22 \pm 0.15$ | $0.27 \pm 0.19$ | $0.32 \pm 0.21$ | $0.19 \pm 0.16$ |
| Gauss-GP5n | $0.03 \pm 0.05$ | $0.09 \pm 0.10$ | $0.18 \pm 0.12$ | $0.24 \pm 0.14$ | $0.30 \pm 0.13$ | $0.17 \pm 0.11$ |
| Gauss-GP7n | $0.02 \pm 0.04$ | $0.07 \pm 0.07$ | $0.14 \pm 0.10$ | $0.20 \pm 0.11$ | $0.24 \pm 0.09$ | $0.13 \pm 0.08$ |
| Gauss-GP9n | $0.02 \pm 0.03$ | $0.05 \pm 0.06$ | $0.10 \pm 0.07$ | $0.17 \pm 0.09$ | $0.20 \pm 0.08$ | $0.11 \pm 0.07$ |
| kNN-IP3o | $0.01 \pm 0.04$ | $0.04 \pm 0.08$ | $0.16 \pm 0.12$ | $0.29 \pm 0.15$ | $0.40 \pm 0.16$ | $0.18 \pm 0.12$ |
| kNN-IP5o | $0.01 \pm 0.04$ | $0.06 \pm 0.09$ | $0.18 \pm 0.13$ | $0.30 \pm 0.15$ | $0.44 \pm 0.18$ | $0.20 \pm 0.13$ |
| kNN-IP7o | $0.02 \pm 0.04$ | $0.07 \pm 0.09$ | $0.19 \pm 0.13$ | $0.31 \pm 0.16$ | $0.45 \pm 0.17$ | $0.21 \pm 0.13$ |
| kNN-IP9o | $0.02 \pm 0.05$ | $0.08 \pm 0.10$ | $0.19 \pm 0.13$ | $0.32 \pm 0.17$ | $0.45 \pm 0.17$ | $0.21 \pm 0.13$ |
| kNN-IP3n | $0.01 \pm 0.04$ | $0.06 \pm 0.08$ | $0.19 \pm 0.13$ | $0.32 \pm 0.16$ | $0.45 \pm 0.19$ | $0.20 \pm 0.13$ |
| kNN-IP5n | $0.02 \pm 0.04$ | $0.07 \pm 0.10$ | $0.21 \pm 0.14$ | $0.36 \pm 0.16$ | $0.49 \pm 0.18$ | $0.23 \pm 0.13$ |
| kNN-IP7n | $0.02 \pm 0.05$ | $0.09 \pm 0.10$ | $0.22 \pm 0.14$ | $0.36 \pm 0.16$ | $0.49 \pm 0.17$ | $0.23 \pm 0.13$ |
| kNN-IP9n | $0.02 \pm 0.05$ | $0.09 \pm 0.11$ | $0.23 \pm 0.14$ | $0.36 \pm 0.16$ | $0.48 \pm 0.17$ | $0.24 \pm 0.13$ |
| kNN-GP3o | $0.02 \pm 0.05$ | $0.08 \pm 0.10$ | $0.21 \pm 0.14$ | $0.34 \pm 0.17$ | $0.46 \pm 0.20$ | $0.22 \pm 0.14$ |
| kNN-GP5o | $0.02 \pm 0.05$ | $0.09 \pm 0.11$ | $0.22 \pm 0.15$ | $0.37 \pm 0.17$ | $0.49 \pm 0.20$ | $0.24 \pm 0.14$ |
| kNN-GP7o | $0.02 \pm 0.05$ | $0.09 \pm 0.12$ | $0.23 \pm 0.15$ | $0.38 \pm 0.18$ | $0.49 \pm 0.19$ | $0.24 \pm 0.15$ |
| kNN-GP9o | $0.02 \pm 0.06$ | $0.09 \pm 0.12$ | $0.23 \pm 0.15$ | $0.37 \pm 0.18$ | $0.49 \pm 0.19$ | $0.24 \pm 0.14$ |
| kNN-GP3n | $0.02 \pm 0.04$ | $0.07 \pm 0.09$ | $0.19 \pm 0.13$ | $0.34 \pm 0.17$ | $0.46 \pm 0.20$ | $0.22 \pm 0.14$ |
| kNN-GP5n | $0.02 \pm 0.05$ | $0.08 \pm 0.10$ | $0.22 \pm 0.15$ | $0.38 \pm 0.18$ | $0.50 \pm 0.19$ | $0.24 \pm 0.14$ |
| kNN-GP7n | $0.02 \pm 0.05$ | $0.09 \pm 0.11$ | $0.23 \pm 0.15$ | $0.39 \pm 0.18$ | $0.51 \pm 0.19$ | $0.25 \pm 0.15$ |
| kNN-GP9n | $0.02 \pm 0.05$ | $0.09 \pm 0.12$ | $0.23 \pm 0.15$ | $0.38 \pm 0.18$ | $0.50 \pm 0.18$ | $0.25 \pm 0.14$ |
| H08b-07w | $0.01 \pm 0.04$ | $0.02 \pm 0.05$ | $0.04 \pm 0.06$ | $0.13 \pm 0.11$ | $0.22 \pm 0.17$ | $0.08 \pm 0.10$ |
| H08b-11w | $0.01 \pm 0.04$ | $0.02 \pm 0.04$ | $0.06 \pm 0.06$ | $0.15 \pm 0.12$ | $0.22 \pm 0.15$ | $0.09 \pm 0.09$ |
| H08b-15w | $0.01 \pm 0.03$ | $0.03 \pm 0.04$ | $0.07 \pm 0.06$ | $0.14 \pm 0.12$ | $0.20 \pm 0.14$ | $0.09 \pm 0.09$ |
| H08b-19w | $0.01 \pm 0.03$ | $0.03 \pm 0.04$ | $0.07 \pm 0.06$ | $0.13 \pm 0.11$ | $0.19 \pm 0.12$ | $0.09 \pm 0.08$ |
| H16b-07w | $0.02 \pm 0.05$ | $0.05 \pm 0.07$ | $0.09 \pm 0.08$ | $0.20 \pm 0.12$ | $0.29 \pm 0.14$ | $0.13 \pm 0.10$ |
| H16b-11w | $0.02 \pm 0.05$ | $0.05 \pm 0.07$ | $0.13 \pm 0.10$ | $0.24 \pm 0.15$ | $0.32 \pm 0.15$ | $0.15 \pm 0.11$ |
| H16b-15w | $0.02 \pm 0.04$ | $0.06 \pm 0.07$ | $0.13 \pm 0.11$ | $0.22 \pm 0.15$ | $0.29 \pm 0.13$ | $0.14 \pm 0.11$ |
| H16b-19w | $0.02 \pm 0.04$ | $0.06 \pm 0.08$ | $0.12 \pm 0.10$ | $0.20 \pm 0.14$ | $0.27 \pm 0.12$ | $0.14 \pm 0.10$ |
| H32b-07w | $0.01 \pm 0.04$ | $0.03 \pm 0.06$ | $0.08 \pm 0.08$ | $0.18 \pm 0.11$ | $0.27 \pm 0.12$ | $0.12 \pm 0.09$ |
| H32b-11w | $0.01 \pm 0.04$ | $0.05 \pm 0.07$ | $0.13 \pm 0.11$ | $0.25 \pm 0.15$ | $0.34 \pm 0.14$ | $0.15 \pm 0.11$ |
| H32b-15w | $0.02 \pm 0.04$ | $0.06 \pm 0.08$ | $0.14 \pm 0.12$ | $0.26 \pm 0.16$ | $0.33 \pm 0.14$ | $0.16 \pm 0.11$ |
| H32b-19w | $0.02 \pm 0.04$ | $0.07 \pm 0.09$ | $0.15 \pm 0.12$ | $0.25 \pm 0.15$ | $0.31 \pm 0.13$ | $0.16 \pm 0.11$ |
| kNN-GP7n-c1 | $0.02 \pm 0.04$ | $0.09 \pm 0.10$ | $0.22 \pm 0.15$ | $0.39 \pm 0.18$ | $0.52 \pm 0.21$ | $0.25 \pm 0.15$ |
| kNN-GP7n-c2 | $0.02 \pm 0.04$ | $0.08 \pm 0.10$ | $0.22 \pm 0.15$ | $0.39 \pm 0.19$ | $0.52 \pm 0.23$ | $0.25 \pm 0.16$ |
| kNN-GP7n-c3 | $0.02 \pm 0.04$ | $0.07 \pm 0.09$ | $0.21 \pm 0.14$ | $0.38 \pm 0.19$ | $0.50 \pm 0.24$ | $0.24 \pm 0.16$ |
| kNN-GP7n-c4 | $0.01 \pm 0.03$ | $0.04 \pm 0.04$ | $0.17 \pm 0.10$ | $0.32 \pm 0.16$ | $0.43 \pm 0.21$ | $0.19 \pm 0.13$ |
| kNN-GP9n-c1 | $0.02 \pm 0.05$ | $0.09 \pm 0.11$ | $0.24 \pm 0.15$ | $0.40 \pm 0.18$ | $0.52 \pm 0.21$ | $0.25 \pm 0.15$ |
| kNN-GP9n-c2 | $0.02 \pm 0.04$ | $0.09 \pm 0.10$ | $0.23 \pm 0.15$ | $0.40 \pm 0.19$ | $0.54 \pm 0.23$ | $0.26 \pm 0.16$ |
| kNN-GP9n-c3 | $0.01 \pm 0.04$ | $0.08 \pm 0.09$ | $0.23 \pm 0.14$ | $0.39 \pm 0.19$ | $0.52 \pm 0.23$ | $0.24 \pm 0.16$ |
| kNN-GP9n-c4 | $0.01 \pm 0.03$ | $0.05 \pm 0.05$ | $0.18 \pm 0.11$ | $0.34 \pm 0.17$ | $0.46 \pm 0.22$ | $0.21 \pm 0.14$ |

**Table 6.7:** Performance of different appearance models on prostate US images for all resolutions $R_0$ (original resolution) to $R_4$ (four times down-sampled). Profile models are labeled as intensity (IP) or gradient profile (GP), followed by their length and an 'o' for original values or 'n' for normalized values. Histogram models are labeled by their number of bins ('b') and the width of the region they are collected in ('w'). For the clustered models, the clustering strategy is given as cl1 to cl4 – see the text for details. All results are given as mean and standard deviation.

| Resolution | Convergence criterion | $\gamma$ | $\Delta$ |
|---|---|---|---|
| 4 | $d_{max} < 0.3$ mm | - | 1 |
| 3 | $I = 200$ | 0.01 | 1 |
| 2 | $I = 200$ | 0.02 | 2 |

**Table 6.8:** Parameter values used in various phases of prostate segmentation. A hyphen '-' for $\gamma$ signifies that the force equilibrium scheme was not used and the surface was restricted to the SSM.

| Measure | Def | App-PW | No-OS | No-FD | App-Std |
|---|---|---|---|---|---|
| VOE [%] | $16.6 \pm 10.2$ | $16.1 \pm 10.0$ | $24.0 \pm 10.0$ | $16.4 \pm 10.1$ | $21.9 \pm 10.0$ |
| RVD [%] | $5.2 \pm 23.9$ | $3.1 \pm 23.0$ | $-12.9 \pm 13.2$ | $5.5 \pm 23.2$ | $-3.3 \pm 13.4$ |
| ASD [mm] | $1.2 \pm 1.0$ | $1.1 \pm 1.0$ | $1.7 \pm 0.8$ | $1.2 \pm 1.0$ | $1.6 \pm 0.8$ |
| RMSSD [mm] | $1.7 \pm 1.4$ | $1.6 \pm 1.4$ | $2.4 \pm 1.0$ | $1.7 \pm 1.4$ | $2.2 \pm 1.1$ |
| MSD [mm] | $6.7 \pm 3.6$ | $6.2 \pm 3.3$ | $8.5 \pm 6.6$ | $6.6 \pm 3.8$ | $8.0 \pm 3.2$ |

**Table 6.9:** Final segmentation results for the prostate for various search strategies.

### Initialization

For the model simplification step, a maximum geodesic distance of $r = 1$ around deleted landmarks was chosen, which reduced the shape model to 126 points. The global search was then conducted in the 4 times down-sampled images $R_4$, for which the employed appearance model also showed the best performance.

Using the same parameter sets as for the other two applications, the performance of the genetic algorithm was evaluated on the first cross-validation set (i.e. 5 test images). Results are given in Fig. 6.21 and show (apart from some exceptions) mostly level graphs. Finally, it was opted to use the following parameter set for the full evaluation: 5 shape parameters to optimize, using a population of 500 individuals over 20 iterations, $\sigma_0 = 0.4$ and $\sigma_{20} = 0.05$ (corresponding to $\sigma = 0.9$), speed of convergence $v = 5$ and perturbation translation factor $\sigma_{trans} = 2$. On a standard PC, the algorithm needed approximately 1 minute and 10 seconds to find a suitable initialization of the SSM in a new image.

### Iterative search

Looking at the extremely low performance of the appearance model in higher resolutions (i.e. $R_0$ and $R_1$), it was decided to use a relatively simple multi-resolution strategy using the lower resolution images exclusively.

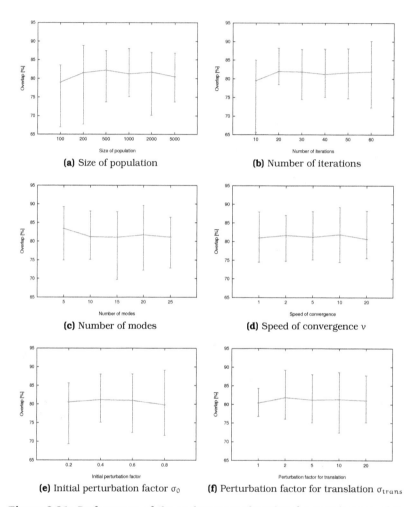

**(a)** Size of population

**(b)** Number of iterations

**(c)** Number of modes

**(d)** Speed of convergence $\nu$

**(e)** Initial perturbation factor $\sigma_0$

**(f)** Perturbation factor for translation $\sigma_{trans}$

**Figure 6.21:** Performance of the evolutionary algorithm for initialization of the prostate model with various parameter sets. For each parameter value, the mean volumetric overlap is given, with error bars spanning the distance from lowest to highest overlap among the five test images.

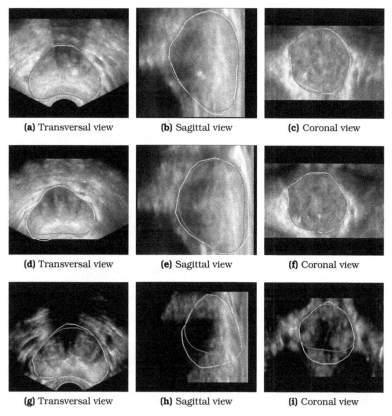

**Figure 6.22:** Selected slices of segmentation results on different prostate US images: the result of the presented search algorithm is displayed in red, the manually traced reference contour in green. Top row (a–c): image representing the $Q_{0.05}$ quantile of average surface distances – one of the best segmentations. Center row (d–f): image representing the median of average surface distances – an average result. Bottom row (g–i): image representing the $Q_{0.95}$ quantile of average surface distances – one of the failed segmentations.

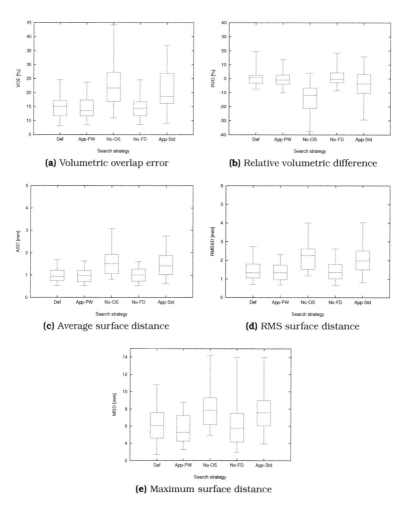

(a) Volumetric overlap error

(b) Relative volumetric difference

(c) Average surface distance

(d) RMS surface distance

(e) Maximum surface distance

**Figure 6.23:** Performance of different iterative search strategies for prostate US images. Box-plots show the median and the surrounding quartiles of the specific quality measure over all 45 images, with the whiskers indicating 5% and 95% quantiles. Results are shown for the developed default algorithm (Def), performance-weighted appearance models (App-PW), no optimal surface detection (No-OS), no free deformation (No-FD) and a standard Gaussian appearance model (App-Std).

As the prostate shapes feature even less variation than the lung, different convergence criteria should not play a high influence. $R_4$ was chosen as resolution for the first phase, followed by two phases in $R_3$ and $R_2$, respectively. Table 6.8 lists the employed parameters for all phases.

As for the other two applications, internal forces were set constant to $\alpha = 0.125$ and $\beta = 0.25$. Restricting the shape model to the first 8 modes of variation, 90% of the total variance could be captured. Again, external forces were evaluated every 10 iterations and 6 probes were taken on each side of the surface. Due to the low voxel spacing, the distance between two probes was set to $d_p = 0.125$ mm in $R_0$. Default setting was not including weighted appearance models.

Visual examples of segmentation quality for the default search strategy are shown in Fig. 6.22, which shows the detected contours in comparison to manual references for three different cases. The quantitative results for the default search strategy and the four variants (weighted appearance models, no optimal surface detection, no free deformation and standard appearance model) are given in Fig. 6.23. In the last variant, a Gaussian normalized gradient profile of length 9 was used as appearance model. Overall, the version with free deformation, optimal surface detection and appearance weighting delivered the best results with an average surface distance of 1.1 mm and an overlap error of 16.1%. On average, the iterative search required 40 seconds for one image.

### 6.3.5 Performance index verification

The final prostate experiment was the correlation of the calculated appearance model performance indices $\xi$ with real-world segmentation results. Weighting factors for $\bar{\xi}$ were adjusted according to the search strategy for the prostate (as given in Table 6.8), which resulted in:

$$\bar{\xi} = \frac{1}{28} \left( 4\xi(R_2) + 8\xi(R_3) + 16\xi(R_4) \right) \tag{6.3}$$

Figure 6.8 shows the relation between this weighted performance index and the obtained segmentation result. The Pearson correlation coefficient between the two variables is $r = 0.83$.

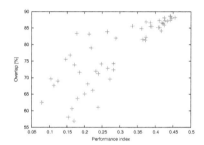

**Figure 6.24:** Correlation between the average performance index $\bar{\xi}$ and the quality of the corresponding segmentation for the prostate US data. To estimate the quality of segmentation, five images were segmented for each appearance model, the volumetric overlaps with the references were calculated and averaged.

# 7 Discussion

> *The truth is rarely pure and never simple.*
>
> — Oscar Wilde, "The Importance of Being Earnest" (1895)

In this chapter, results of the presented experiments are discussed in detail. The ordering is the same as in the previous chapter, first covering the liver in Sec. 7.1, the lung in Sec. 7.2, and finally the prostate in Sec. 7.3. In addition, general aspects of this work which concern all applications are discussed in Sec. 7.4.

## 7.1 Evaluation on the liver (CT)

### 7.1.1 Shape model construction

Out of the three chosen applications, the liver was the most challenging to build a shape model for. First, the basic liver shape itself is comparatively complex with its pronounced edges and the anatomy of two lobes defined by the internal vessel systems. Second, the used training shapes featured by far the largest variations. This is not only obvious from the visualization of the different samples in Fig. 6.1, but also from the compactness results in Fig. 6.2, which shows the average variation per landmark. For the entire training set (i.e. using all available modes), this variance is around 60 mm – as a comparison, the similar-sized left lung lobe features only an average variance of 17 mm per landmark.

Taking into account the enormous variation, the detected correspondences seem quite prudent. The coordinate grid in Fig. 6.1 shows the same colors for regions that would intuitively be regarded as corresponding. However, there are some exceptions, most notable the fourth sample in the first row. Here, one problem becomes immediately apparent by looking at the extreme distortion of the coordinate grid at the upper left side. The strong distortion indicates that the optimization algorithm heavily modified the parameterization in this region, and without landmark reconfiguration the area would

feature very few landmark points. A second problem can only be recognized knowing the original anatomy of this case, where the elongated part is directed towards the viewer, not towards the top. In the used implementation, the optimizer allows rotating all training samples to the orientation which results in the lowest cost function – these rotations could also be limited to the vertical axis, potentially producing better results. All in all, these distortion problems only occur for a very limited number of training samples and did not impede the construction of a valid shape model. The extracted modes of variation of Fig. 6.3 produce realistic shapes which appear in similar form in the training set as well.

For quantitative comparison between three different variants of construction of the shape model (Fig. 6.2), the results are varied. From an earlier experiment with less training samples [102], it was expected that the continuous landmark reconfiguration scheme would produce significantly better results than the other two methods. As it is, generalization of the continuously reconfigured model is better in the interesting region of 10–15 modes (which capture 90–95% of the total variance). However, specificity is approximately the same as for the standard model. The model which is only reconfigured once reaches the best results for specificity, although all differences are only minimal. For the compactness measure, the reconfigured models score both significantly worse than the standard model. However, as explained above, compactness simply describes the average variance per landmark, and as the standard optimization leads to placing less landmarks in the highly varying shapes, the average variance is lower (as already observed in Sec. 3.5). An interesting revelation from the generalization plot is that utilizing the full number of modes, the volumetric error for the leave-one-out test resides around 9%. This high value indicates that the 45 training samples used here are not enough to capture the large variance of the population, and that additional deformation during segmentation should result in significant improvements.

### 7.1.2 Appearance models

Box-plots in Fig. 6.4 offer a good overview of the average performance of the various appearance models. Starting with the classical Gaussian profile models, the first surprise is that shorter profiles constantly reach better results than longer profiles. One would have expected the opposite circumstance, which has also been described in the first quantitative evaluation of appearance models by Cootes and Taylor [34]. In that experiment, the au-

thors scored the appearance models according to the performance reached by a series of ASM segmentations – arguably a more reliable estimate than the presented simulated search. However, the performance index verification conducted later on confirmed these first findings (except for the normalized gradient profile – more on that in Sec. 7.1.4). One possible explanation for this effect is that the amount of training data is not sufficient to build a reliable appearance model with a longer profile length – as larger profiles equal an increase of dimension of the sample space, they require more data to deliver comparable model accuracy. Another reason could be that the non-linearities of the training data show through more prominently with extended length profiles, which would explain why this effect is much less pronounced with non-linear profiles. For the Gaussian appearance models, normalization does not improve performance of intensity profiles, but yields noticeably better results for gradient profiles.

All tested non-linear models reach better, in some cases significantly better results than their Gaussian counterparts. This can partly be attributed to the non-linearities in the data which cannot be captured by Gaussian models. Another reason is that the kNN-classifier, trained on boundary and background data, can differentiate more reliably between these two distributions. Although the effect is not as strong as for the Gaussian models, shorter profiles outperform the larger variants in some cases. As in the previous case, this outcome can be attributed to the lack of sufficient training data.

The local histogram models could not unfold their strengths in this application and reach similar scores as in the Gaussian profiles. Interestingly, performance breaks down drastically when using 32 bins, and even 16 bins do not reach the scores of 8 bins. Since 32 bins do work well for other kinds of images (as the lung MRI data), the problem cannot consist of the histogram not acquiring sufficient samples. Rather, it seems as if the characteristic gray-value differences on the liver boundary can better be captured at a rougher intensity scale.

Clustering the chosen non-linear models led to a major boost in performance, especially for the rougher resolution levels. At these rougher resolutions, the profiles span a larger part of the image, which leads to more variation. Increasing the amount of training samples (which is what the clustering efficiently does) permits to model this increased variation more reliably. More training samples also allow a higher dimension of the sample

space, which explains why the 7 pixel long profiles shows a better performance than the 5 pixel version in the clustered variant.

### 7.1.3 Segmentation

The first experiment (Sec. 6.1.4) was designed to evaluate the effects of parameter changes for the evolutionary algorithm, expecting that a fair amount of troubleshooting would be required to obtain stable results. As the outcome in Fig. 6.5 reveals, the employed algorithm is surprisingly robust to individual parameter changes: only extreme variations lead to significant changes in the outcome. To interpret these results, the minimum overlap plays a very important role, almost as much as the mean: one failed initialization will also lead to a failed local search, while several mediocre initializations might well be recovered in that subsequent step.

As an initial attempt revealed, it was not possible to combine the individual best parameters into one best set: although the initialization runs reasonably stable with a small population or with few iterations, both taken together impede the performance noticeably. Because of the high variation of the shape model, increasing the number of modes lead to a better overlap for the initialization. However, as the subsequent local search was run with 10 modes, it did not make sense to use more than these 10 in the first step.

In general, the evolutionary algorithm delivered reasonable results for the liver, and the subsequent local search could start without further user interaction. The required computation time though – up to 6 minutes – is almost twice as much as needed for the local search and could still be improved.

The final search using the deformable model produced generally favorable results. Previous publications about liver segmentation reached an average surface distance of 2 mm (utilizing a deformable model without shape constraints [216]) and 2.3 mm (utilizing a statistical shape model without free deformation [137]). In contrast, the method presented here yielded an average surface distance of 1.5 mm. For further comparison purposes, segmentations created by a second rater for ten of the employed images resulted in an average volumetric overlap error of VOE=6.4% and an average surface distance of ASD=1 mm [255]. The results obtained with the presented automated method are still a step away from these numbers, but taking only the best 80% of segmentations into account, errors decrease to a VOE of 6.8% and an ASD of 1.2 mm. These numbers are sufficiently close

to employ the automated method for clinical tasks, especially when 100% accuracy is not required. One example of such an application would be a quick 3D visualization of the vessel systems inside the liver, which depends on a rough mask of the liver tissue. Segmentations as shown in the upper two rows of Fig. 6.6 would be perfectly suitable for that purpose.

From the results in Table 6.3, the advantage of additional variability that was added with the deformable mesh is clearly visible. As the used CT images offer a sound signal-to-noise ratio, the optimal surface detection yielded only slight improvements for this application, and it should only be applied in the later phases of the search. Initial tests using the optimal surface detection directly from resolution $R_4$ even resulted in decreased performance: for some images, relatively large boundary adjustments were required in this step, and the optimal surface detection actually stabilized the model too much.

High variation of the liver model makes the local search very susceptible to used multi-resolution strategy. A reasonable fit in the rougher resolutions is essential for a successful segmentation, as errors made in $R_4$ or $R_3$ cannot be corrected later on. An example of a segmentation that failed for this reason is shown in the lower row of Fig. 6.6, where the boundary locked to the kidney at the very beginning of the segmentation and remained there until the final result. To prevent these errors, care has to be taken that the search does not switch to the next phase before the model has detected the correct structures. In some rare cases, when the model was too far away from the true boundary, self-intersections of the deformable mesh occured. These loops in the surface, once they emerged, could not be corrected either. Overall, 90% of variation covered by the used 10 modes are probably a lower limit for the liver: using more modes in the beginning would improve initialization and segmentation in the rougher resolutions, potentially preventing some of the ocurring problems.

It was also surprising to see the low performance of the standard Gaussian profile model in the final test. The performance index indicated that the chosen model was problematic, but it resulted as virtually unusable for segmentation. Again, this can be attributed to the complex shape of the liver and its variable surroundings: if an appearance model cannot initially lock onto the true contours, the segmentation will generally fail entirely.

### 7.1.4 Performance Index verification

The Pearson correlation coefficient of $r = 0.66$ between the theoretical performance index $\xi$ and the obtained real-world results is not as high as originally expected. Further examining the graph in Fig. 6.8, it is obvious that there is a correlation between the two variables, albeit not a linear one. Especially for the lowest performance indices, the segmentation results break down abruptly. As noted before, this behaviour can be explained by the complexity of the segmentation task. A more severe problem is that for $\xi$ between 0.2 and 0.4 (the Gaussian profile models), correlation seems very low. After closer inspection it was revealed that the segmentation performance of the normalized gradient models is far better than their performance index indicates. This problem is discussed in more detail in Sec. 7.4 of this chapter. A positive result of the experiment is that all appearance models with high $\xi$ also reached excellent segmentation results. Therefore, chosing appearance models according to the calculated performance indices seems a valid procedure for this segmentation task.

## 7.2 Evaluation on the lung (MRI)

### 7.2.1 Shape model construction

The most interesting aspect when constructing the SSM of the left lung lobe was how well the presented approach would cope with training sets of larger size. The results were positively surprising: The ability to construct a shape model from over 160 training samples in only 50 hours means that there are no restrictions by computational constraints when enlarging shape models with new data. Model construction was much faster (relative to the number of samples) than for the liver, basically due to the following reasons: first, training meshes for the lung were significantly simpler than for the liver (both in terms of vertex count and shape), second, less landmarks were used for the lung, and third, training shapes for the lung were much more similar to each other, which required less iterations to optimize correspondences.

As far as it can be judged from the common coordinate-grids in Fig. 6.9, the final point correspondences are very accurate. Contrary to the liver samples, there were no distortion problems with the parameterizations. The largest modes of variation in Fig. 6.11 also appear very realistic: features are well-kept and variations look natural. As can be seen in Fig. 6.10, the

generalization ability of the lung model is significantly better than for the liver. Using the maximum number of modes, the volumetric overlap error is around 5% – given the low resolution of the lung images, this is a very good result[1]. The reason for the noisy specificity graph is that only 100 random shapes per mode were generated to estimate each number (instead of 10,000 used for the other applications) in order to keep the computational costs down – due to the high number of required shape comparisons, specificity is the most time-consuming measure to calculate.

## 7.2.2 Appearance models

When looking at the box-plots in Fig 6.12, we notice the same effect as for the livers: the longer the Gaussian profiles are, the more their performance decreases. The verification experiment conducted later confirmed this trend for the unnormalized profiles, the real-world performance of the normalized profiles however stayed approximately the same for longer versions.

Non-linear models deliver excellent performance in all variations, as the large amount of training images provides a sound basis for the employed kNN-classifier. Subsequent clustering only slightly improves the values, which is also a hint that the training data is not a problem for this application.

As with the liver, the histogram models showed similar performance as the Gaussian profiles. Apparently, analyzing larger regions of data is not much of an advantage for the low resolution of the lung images when detecting the boundary.

Another effect that can be attributed to the low resolution is the surprisingly good performance at the original resolution $R_0$ (see Table 6.4). In this application, almost 4 mm separate two adjacent voxels in $R_0$, and changes in tissue are much more prominent at this scale than at the submillimeter spacing of the liver CT images. Down-sampling the MRI data more than twice did not seem prudent under these conditions, as only a dozen voxels would remain along the shortest axis of the image. Not surprisingly, performance values start to decrease with $R_3$ for all appearance models, even for the clustered non-linear ones. This is also a clue for the optimal resolution to be used for initialization, as we will see in the next section.

---

[1]For objects comprised of fewer voxels, small deviations result in larger overlap errors than for bigger objects.

### 7.2.3 Segmentation

Some initial tests with different resolutions for the evolutionary algorithm confirmed the performance data from the appearance models, and thus $R_2$ was chosen as resolution for this step. Varying the different parameters of the algorithm had only marginal effects, as can be seen in Fig. 6.13. Especially in comparison with the large differences between individual images (displayed by the error bars), the observed changes are minimal. These findings show that the evolutionary search is very robust with regard to its internal parameters.

The main reason for the varying successes when initializing the model on different images, is the specific variability of the lung which originates from the motion during the breathing cycle. The principal variation is the up-and-down movement of the lung base, which means that it is possible to perfectly fit the model to all side walls and the top of the lung (yielding very high fitting values), but missing the base. An example for such a case is shown in Fig. 6.14 (i). The time required for an initialization (approx. 2 minutes) is noticeably less than for the liver, but it is still a multiple of the amount required for the iterative search.

Due to the low resolution of the input images and the small number of phases used in the multi-resolution framework, the iterative search was completed very quickly. The obtained results, listed in Table 6.6, are reasonably good, especially considering the low resolution: the average surface distance of 2.3 mm already reaches sub-voxel accuracy. As the primary goal of the lung segmentation is its use for volumetry, the relative volumetric distance is of special interest for this application. While 2.3% seems like an excellent result, the decisive value here is the standard deviation, which could still be improved.

In the same table, it is interesting to note that there is apparently no advantage in using the free deformation in this application: the performance increases if the search is conducted without free deformation. This is due to the high number of training samples and the resulting large number of modes available for this model. Note that the default search was conducted with 15 modes of variation, but the variant without free deformation was run with the full number of 145 modes.

Another observation is that (contrary to the liver experiments) the standard appearance model reaches competitive performance, almost on the same level as the non-linear kNN model used in the default variant. Even leaving out the optimal surface detection does not result in any degradation

of performance. As in the previous case, these results can be attributed to the large number of training samples and the excellent performance of the appearance models. If these are accurate, then there is no need for a robust search such as the optimal surface detection offers. However, the weighting of appearance models led to noticeable improvements (Table 6.6). This can be explained after looking at the box-plots displaying the appearance performance in Fig. 6.12 (f). Although the average performance of the used appearance models is very high, the lower whiskers still decrease to $\xi = 0.2$, and down-weighting these inferior models seems generally advisable.

As mentioned above, the largest errors encountered during the lung segmentation ocurred at the base of the lung lobe: wrong initial shapes could generally not be corrected during the iterative search. An enhancement that might improve segmentation results would be to take information of the time during the breathing cycle into account by generating a 4D model (i.e. 3D + time). With the additional information, the shape model would learn when the lung base is supposed to be at which location, and misalignments in that area could be prevented.

### 7.2.4 Performance index verification

The results of the correlation experiment in Fig. 6.16 look very similar to the output of the corresponding experiment on the liver data There are three outliers at the low end which weaken the correlation coefficient, and correlation for the Gaussian models ($\xi \in [0.2, 0.4]$) is relatively weak. However, the best-rated appearance models deliver the most accurate segmentation results again, which validates the use of the performance indices for selecting an appropriate appearance model.

## 7.3 Evaluation on the prostate (US)

### 7.3.1 Shape model construction

Among the three objects of interest evaluated in this thesis, the prostate was the one with the simplest shape, and no problems were expected for the construction of the geometrical model. The bean-like shapes resulted in virtually distortion-free parameterizations, as can be seen in Fig. 6.17. As the initial conformal parameterizations already showed reasonably good correspondences, landmarks did not require major adjustments and the optimization converged in a very short time. Due to the small changes in

landmark locations, landmark reconfiguration did not involve a significant effect, and the standard model (built without it) was chosen for the subsequent steps.

As far as can be judged from the smooth shapes in Fig. 6.17, the detected correspondences are accurate and prove that the used optimization approach does not require distinctive features to find correspondences. The extracted modes of variation displayed in Fig. 6.19 seem sensible and correspond to samples observed in the training set. Regarding the quantitative evaluation in Fig. 6.19, the generalization error at the maximum number of modes is quite low at 5%, even with the relatively low number of training samples. This indicates a high amount of systematic variation in the training data, an interpretation that is also supported by the steep graph of compactness. Obviously, a large part of total variation is concentrated in the first modes, which is an ideal condition for building a shape model.

### 7.3.2 Appearance models

Building a good appearance model was the most challenging part for the prostate due to the low signal-to-noise ratio of the ultrasound images. As for the other two applications, the spacing for the profile models was chosen according to the spacing of the typical input image. In the case of the prostate however, this strategy did not work out well. As mentioned in Sec. 6.3.1, all input images were preprocessed with a large 7x7x7 median filter mask to remove excessive noise. At that scale, no details hinting at the boundary could be resolved, which led to performance indices close to zero for the original resolution $R_0$ (see Table 6.7). Performance only increases to usable values at $R_2$ and above, suggesting that it might have been more appropriate to down-sample the original data in the beginning and use larger profile spacings.

To compare the performance of different appearance models, the boxplots in Fig. 6.20 are more difficult to interpret. As they display the combined results from all resolutions (with $R_0$ and $R_1$ delivering values close to zero for all models), differences in performance are not as obvious. Listing the results for each resolution separately, Table 6.7 is more suitable for an exact analysis. Taking a closer look at the numbers reveals the following general picture: local histograms show a performance comparable to Gaussian profile models, while non-linear profiles using the kNN classifier reach significantly better values. The clustered versions of the non-linear models improve only marginally over the original versions, which is surprising

given that the prostate boundary appears to be quite suitable for clustering and there is very little training data available for the unclustered versions.

### 7.3.3 Segmentation

The evaluation of different parameter sets for the evolutionary algorithm produced similar results as for the other two applications. Apart from some extreme variations, the initialization delivered a very stable performance with an average overlap around 80% (Fig. 6.21). The main reason for this comparatively high value is the relatively large size of the prostate in the US images (see Fig. 6.22): The structure lies very close to the image boundaries on three sides, and with little space for translation, large overlaps are almost guaranteed. One other point to be considered here is that at the roughest resolution $R_4$ (in which the initialization was run), many boundary profiles leave the image at their outer ends. As outside locations return an intensity of zero, the image boundary features a prominent gradient which is also captured by the appearance models. This results in the appearance models implicitly learning the common distances from prostate to image boundary. If the prostate is not located at the expected position due to variant image acquisition, this dependency leads to failures during the initialization.

When analyzing the results of the different variants of the iterative search in Fig. 6.23, it becomes obvious which extensions to the conventional search are required to deliver satisfying results for this application, namely optimal surface detection and non-linear appearance models. Given the low signal-to-noise ratio of the US images, this result was to be expected: the optimal surface detection supresses the effect of outliers and makes the entire search more robust, whilst a well-performing appearance model prevents outliers from the start. The free deformation, on the other hand, did not involve a positive effect. Leaving it out and using the full set of constrained modes even slightly improved the results. This effect is due to the low amount of variations encountered in the prostate model, which is also indicated by the good compactness values.

A slightly surprising result is that the appearance weighting did not lead to higher improvements of the segmentation results. According to the boxplots in Fig. 6.20, there are at least some reliable appearance models ($\xi >$ 0.8) that should have a higher impact when using weighting.

Comparing the three applications, the prostate segmentation subjectively delivered the most impressive results. For the untrained eye, the prostate

boundary is often not recognizable in the US images (see Fig. 6.22 for some examples), yet the shape model managed to detect it accurately. The objective evaluation measures listed in Table 6.9 support this impression: a volumetric overlap error of 16.1% and an average surface distance of 1.1 mm are acceptable results, considering that these numbers also include the failed segmentations. Calculating the mean over the most successful 80% of segmentations results in a VOE of 12.8% and an ASD of 0.9 mm. Incidentally, these are almost exactly the same values as determined in a reproducibility study, in which the same human operator had to segment the same prostate images twice, with a time-span of several weeks in between. This means that the presented segmenation approach delivers human-like performance in the vast majority of cases for this application.

### 7.3.4 Performance index verification

The experiment to verify the developed performance index yielded the highest correlation for the prostate with $r > 0.8$. Although this correlation is still far from perfect, a clear linear relationship between estimated performance and obtained segmentation result is visible in Fig. 6.24. The figure also reveals that the highest-rated models also produce the best segmentations, which validates the selection procedure for the employed appearance models. In the next section, the reasons for this high correlation (relative to the other applications) are discussed in detail.

## 7.4 General discussion

### 7.4.1 Shape model construction

As documented by overlaid coordinate grids and visualization of the principal modes of variation for all examined applications, the developed method for correspondence optimization is able to produce satisfactory results in a reasonable amount of time. However, the real performance of the method can only be determined by a direct comparison with alternative approaches on the same data. These comparisons are hindered by the fact that most algorithms for 3D correspondence detection are not publicly available. To present the gradient descent optimization developed in this thesis at a conference [103], a couple of synthetic and real-life training sets were sent to the University of Manchester to produce results with the original MDL method [52]. As the outcome revealed, the gradient descent method not

only ran several orders of magnitude faster, but also resulted in better values for generalization and specificity[2].

To make the gradient descent correspondence optimization available for other interested researchers, the algorithm was released as open source code for the ITK image analysis framework [101]. People and groups which tested and employed the algorithm so far include:

- Ipek Oguz at the University of North Carolina at Chapel Hill, NC, USA

- Martin Spiegel at the University of Erlangen-Nürnberg, Germany

- Paulette Lieby at National ICT Australia, Australia

- Ekaterina Syrkina at ETH Zürich, Switzerland

- Corné Hoogendoorn at the IT University Copenhague, Denmark

- Defeng Wang at the Chinese University of Hong Kong, China

- Zihua Su at Siemens Corporate Research, Princeton, NJ, USA

### 7.4.2 Appearance models

In all considered applications, the best-performing appearance models were the clustered non-linear profiles. This predominance is attributed to the fact that these models are the only ones from the examined set which are not only trained on boundary appearance, but also on background appearance. Although kNN is a relatively simple classifier, it was able to translate this additional information to much better segmentation results.

Performance of the local histogram model was a bit disappointing overall. Perhaps the $L_1$ distance to the closest sample in the training set is not the optimal cost function here, but some tests with the Earthmover distance suggested by Broadhurst et al. [24] did not result in better performance either. One modification which could boost performance substantially is to employ a kNN-classifier for this model to separate inner and outer histograms, but this is a topic for future work.

---

[2]As these experiments were run on different data sets than the ones presented in Sec. 6, the results are not contained in this thesis.

### 7.4.3 Segmentation

In this thesis, several extensions to the classical SSM search were developed and tested. As it turned out, the effectiveness of these extensions always depends on the specific application. For the liver with its large variability, the additional free deformation was essential for good segmentation results, while it did not result in any improvements for the lung. Similarly, the noisy prostate images could draw maximum benefit from the robust optimal surface detection, which was not as important for the liver.

A good reason for employing the optimal surface detection in any case is that it forms the basis for weighting the appearance costs with the individual performance indices, which lead to improved results for all examined applications. Although other weighting schemes exist for the standard search algorithms, it is not clear if they will peform equally well in this respect.

### 7.4.4 Performance index verification

For all examined applications, performance of the Gaussian profile models did not correlate satisfactorily with the obtained segmentation results. Often the performance index decreased with larger profile sizes, while the accuracy of the corresponding segmentations actually increased. What is the reason for this behaviour of an otherwise well-correlating measure?

The answer to that question is best explained using a simple boundary model with a fixed intensity on the inner side and a fixed intensity on the outer side. Let us assume that the general variation along an intensity profile as extracted from the set of training images is equal for all samples in the profile. When shifting the profile to the outer side of the object, the largest differences occur at the center locations, as positions which describe inner intensity values will be moved out of the object. The amount of induced variation only depends on the range of shifting, not on the length of the profile. However, a given range of shifting has a larger impact on shorter profiles, because differences appear greater relative to the total profile variation. For this reason, fitting costs are rising faster for shorter profiles than for longer ones when shifting, which leads to better performance indices. In practice, this problem is difficult to solve, as the strength of the effect always depends on the used data.

To conclude, the presented performance index is best suited for benchmarking individual landmarks featuring the same model. For this task, it

works extremely well, as the positive results of appearance weighting during search demonstrate. Nevertheless, it can also be used to select the best appearance model from a set of candidates, since a high index (at least for the examined applications) also corresponds to good segmentation results.

# 8 Conclusions

*On two occasions I have been asked,*
*"Pray, Mr. Babbage, if you put into the machine wrong figures,*
*will the right answers come out?" [...]*
*I am not able rightly to apprehend the kind of confusion of ideas*
*that could provoke such a question.*

— Charles Babbage, "Passages from the Life of a Philosopher" (1864)

The problem of segmentation in medical imaging is the major bottleneck for translating advanced computer-based procedures into clinical practice and for making the new technologies available for a larger number of patients. The manual segmentation approach widely used today is too cumbersome, too time-consuming and too expensive to be employed outside of medical studies or specialized niches.

The statistical shape approach presented in this thesis is one step towards the final goal of automating more and more segmentation tasks in the clinic. Although the method does not reach the performance of a human operator on all images, it is able to stand its ground. In case of the prostate segmentation, the most successful 80% of automated segmentations reached the same accuracy as determined in an intra-observer test (the same person segmenting the same images twice), and for the liver the best 80% get close to the values of an inter-observer test (different persons segmenting the same images). No inter- or intra-observer data was available for the lung segmentation, but results here are likely to follow in the same direction.

Having a segmentation method that is able to automatically analyze 80% of images with satisfactory accuracy, the human operator can produce significantly more output than before, as he only needs to approve the majority of cases. And no matter how reliable automated segmentation methods might become, in the foreseeable future there will always be a human operator approving results in clinical practice, even if it is only for legal reasons. Thus, creating automated methods that deliver adequate results

for as much cases as possible is the only viable route to let more patients benefit from modern medical imaging.

This thesis did not present a completely new method for that purpose, but, following a detailed analysis of the current state of the art, it identified problematic points along the entire chain of methods, and presented solutions to these problems. As such, the main contribution of this thesis is a complete system for training, evaluating and employing statistical models of shape and appearance for the purpose of 3D image analysis. The system is trainable without human interaction in reasonable time, it delivers robust, accurate and fast segmentation performance, and it is applicable to a wide range of problems. Thus, all objectives stated in the introduction have been fulfilled.

## 8.1 Summary of contributions

The specific contributions of this thesis are (starting with the highest impact):

1. A novel optimization method to automatically determine correspondences on a set of genus zero shapes, faster and more accurate than previous approaches.

2. The integration of a globally optimal surface detection scheme in an iterative deformable model search, leading to improved robustness of the segmentation.

3. The extension of the constrained shape model search with free deformation based on a deformable model framework with internal forces of tension and rigidity, calculated according to the best fitting shape from the SSM.

4. An evolutionary algorithm for automated model initialization in 3D images.

5. A comparative evaluation of different appearance models and search strategies on a large number of clinical images for three applications.

6. A landmark reconfiguration scheme for the model construction step which leads to smoother surface representations for complex shapes (i.e. when parameterizations feature high distortions).

7. A performance index to evaluate the quality of individual appearance models which can be used as weighting factors during the seach to improve robustness.

8. A comprehensive survey of 3D shape models for medical image analysis, presenting the pricipal directions of research during the last decade.

## 8.2 Future work

A thesis can only follow a limited amount of ideas and directions, and even those can sometimes not be explored until the last detail. Below is a list of future work, arising from the observations in this thesis:

- 3D+t shape models: as discussed in Sec. 7.2.3, models including information about dynamic processes could be of great advantage for applications like lung and heart analysis.

- Hierarchical/combined shape models: there is work on hierarchical SSMs in other groups [202, 195, 57] which would be interesting to integrate with the presented approach. For the liver segmentation, the *V. Cava* could be modeled by a separate SSM, and models of both lung lobes could be combined.

- Histogram-controlled appearance models:  appearance models could be made more specific by performing a histogram analysis of the image as a first step and using the obtained results to chose an appropriate offset for intensity profiles.

- Intersection prevention: to prevent self-intersections of the deformable model, an intersection detection and removal step could be integrated into the local search algorithm. This would be especially beneficial for complex shape models which require a substantial amount of additional free deformation, as the liver examined in this work.

# Bibliography

[1] P. Alliez, M. Meyer, and M. Desbrun. Interactive geometry remeshing. *ACM Transactions on Graphics*, 21(3):347–354, 2002.

[2] P. R. Andresen, F. L. Bookstein, K. Couradsen, B. K. Ersboll, J. L. Marsh, and S. Kreiborg. Surface-bounded growth modeling applied to human mandibles. *IEEE Trans Med Imaging*, 19(11):1053–1063, Nov 2000.

[3] J. Arvo. *Graphics Gems III*, chapter Fast random rotation matrices, pages 117–120. Academic Press, 1992.

[4] J. Bailleul, S. Ruan, D. Bloyet, and B. Romaniuk. Segmentation of anatomical structures from 3D brain MRI using automatically-built statistical shape models. In *Proc ICIP*, volume 4, pages 2741–2744, 24-27 Oct. 2004.

[5] S. Baker and I. Matthews. Equivalence and efficiency of image alignment algorithms. In *Proc IEEE CVPR*, volume 1, pages 1090–1097, 2001.

[6] R. Bansal, L. H. Staib, D. Xu, H. Zhu, and B. S. Peterson. Statistical analyses of brain surfaces using gaussian random fields on 2-D manifolds. *IEEE Trans Med Imaging*, 26(1):46–57, Jan. 2007.

[7] V. Barnett and T. Lewis. *Outliers in statistical data*. Wiley, New York, 1994.

[8] M. Baumhauer, T. Simpfendörfer, R. Schwarz, M. Seitel, B. P. Müller-Stich, C. N. Gutt, J. Rassweiler, H.-P. Meinzer, and I. Wolf. Evaluation of camera pose estimation for enhanced visualization. In *Proc SPIE Medical Imaging 2007: Visualization and Image-Guided Procedures*, volume 6509. SPIE Press, 2007.

[9] G. Behiels, F. Maes, D. Vandermeulen, and P. Suetens. Evaluation of image features and search strategies for segmentation of bone structures in radiographs using active shape models. *Med Image Anal*, 6(1):47–62, Mar 2002.

[10] R. Beichel, H. Bischof, F. Leberl, and M. Sonka. Robust active appearance models and their application to medical image analysis. *IEEE Trans Med Imaging*, 24(9):1151–1169, Sept. 2005.

[11] R. Beichel, G. Gotschuli, E. Sorantin, F. Leberl, and M. Sonka. Diaphragm dome surface segmentation in CT data sets: A 3-D active appearance model approach. In *Proc SPIE Medical Imaging: Image Processing*, volume 4684, pages 475–484, 2002.

[12] P. J. Besl and N. D. McKay. A method for registration of 3-D shapes. *IEEE Trans Pattern Anal Mach Intell*, 14(2):239–256, 1992.

[13] J. M. Blackall, A. P. King, G. P. Penney, A. Adam, and D. J. Hawkes. A statistical model of respiratory motion and deformation of the liver. In *Proc MICCAI*, volume 2208 of *LNCS*, pages 1338–1340. Springer, 2001.

[14] H. Blum. Biological shape and visual science. *J Theor Biol*, 38(2):205–287, Feb 1973.

[15] T. Boettger, T. Kunert, H.-P. Meinzer, and I. Wolf. Interactive constraints for 3D-simplex meshes. In J. M. Fitzpatrick and J. M. Reinhardt, editors, *Proc SPIE Medical Imaging 2005: Image Processing*, volume 5747, pages 1692–1702. SPIE Press, Apr 2005.

[16] F. L. Bookstein. *Morphometric Tools for Landmark Data*. Cambridge University Press, 2003.

[17] J. Bosch, S. Mitchell, B. Lelieveldt, F. Nijland, O. Kamp, M. Sonka, and J. Reiber. Automatic segmentation of echocardiographic sequences by active appearance motion models. *IEEE Trans Med Imaging*, 21(11):1374–1383, Nov. 2002.

[18] Y. Boykov and V. Kolmogorov. An experimental comparison of min-cut/max-flow algorithms for energy minimization in vision. *IEEE Trans Pattern Analysis and Machine Intelligence*, 26(9):1124–1137, 2004.

[19] C. Brechbühler, G. Gerig, and O. Kübler. Parameterization of closed surfaces for 3d shape description. *Comput Vis Image Underst*, 61:154–170, 1995.

[20] M. Brejl and M. Sonka. Object localization and border detection criteria design in edge-based image segmentation: automated learning from examples. *IEEE Trans Med Imaging*, 19(10):973–985, Oct 2000.

[21] A. D. Brett and C. J. Taylor. A method of automated landmark generation for automated 3D PDM construction. *Image Vision Comput*, 18(9):739–748, 1999.

[22] A. D. Brett and C. J. Taylor. Automated construction of 3D shape models using harmonic maps. In *Proc Medical Image Understanding and Analysis*, pages 175–178, 2000.

[23] R. Broadhurst, J. Stough, S. Pizer, and E. Chaney. A statistical appearance model based on intensity quantile histograms. In *Proc IEEE Int Symposium on Biomedical Imaging*, pages 422–425, 6-9 April 2006.

[24] R. E. Broadhurst, J. Stough, S. M. Pizer, and E. L. Chaney. Histogram statistics of local model-relative image regions. In O. F. Olsen, L. Florack, and A. Kuijper, editors, *Proc Deep Structure, Singularities and Computer Vision*, pages 72–83, June 2005.

[25] R. Brunelli and O. Mich. Histograms analysis for image retrieval. *Pattern Recognition*, 34(8):1625–1637, 2001.

[26] J. Cates, P. T. Fletcher, M. A. Styner, M. E. Shenton, and R. T. Whitaker. Shape modeling and analysis with entropy-based particle systems. In N. Karssemeijer and B. P. F. Lelieveldt, editors, *Proc IPMI*, volume 4584 of *LNCS*, pages 333–345. Springer, 2007.

[27] A. Caunce and C. J. Taylor. Building 3D sulcal models using local geometry. *Med Image Anal*, 5:69–80, 2001.

[28] C. S. K. Chan, P. J. Edwards, and D. J. Hawkes. Integration of ultrasound based registration with statistical shape models for computer assisted orthopaedic surgery. In M. Sonka and J. M. Fitzpatrick, editors, *Proc SPIE Medical Imaging: Image Processing*, volume 5032, pages 414–424, San Diego, CA, 2003. SPIE Press.

[29] D. Comaniciu and P. Meer. Mean shift: a robust approach toward feature space analysis. *IEEE Trans Pattern Anal Mach Intell*, 24(5):603–619, May 2002.

[30] T. F. Cootes, G. J. Edwards, and C. J. Taylor. Active appearance models. In H. Burkhardt and B. Neumann, editors, *Proc ECCV*, volume 2, pages 484–498, 1998.

[31] T. F. Cootes, G. J. Edwards, and C. J. Taylor. A comparative evaluation of active appearance model algorithms. In P. Lewis and M. Nixon, editors, *Proc British Machine Vision Conference*, volume 2, pages 680–689, Southampton, UK, Sep 1998. BMVA Press.

[32] T. F. Cootes, G. J. Edwards, and C. J. Taylor. Active appearance models. *IEEE Trans Pattern Anal Mach Intell*, 23(6):681–685, June 2001.

[33] T. F. Cootes and P. Kittipanya-ngam. Comparing variations on the active appearance model algorithm. In *Proc British Machine Vision Conference*, pages 837–846. BMVA Press, September 2002.

[34] T. F. Cootes and C. J. Taylor. Active shape model search using local grey-level models: A quantitative evaluation. In J. Illingworth, editor, *Proc British Machine Vision Conference*, pages 639–648. BMVA Press, 1993.

[35] T. F. Cootes and C. J. Taylor. Using grey-level models to improve active shape model search. In *Proc ICPR*, volume 1, pages 63–67vol.1, 9-13 Oct. 1994.

[36] T. F. Cootes and C. J. Taylor. Combining point distribution models with shape models based on finite-element analysis. *Image Vision Comput*, 13(5):403–409, June 1995.

[37] T. F. Cootes and C. J. Taylor. Data driven refinement of active shape model search. In *Proc British Machine Vision Conference*, pages 383–392. BMVA Press, 1996.

[38] T. F. Cootes and C. J. Taylor. A mixture model for representing shape variation. *Image Vision Comput*, 17(8):567–574, 1999.

[39] T. F. Cootes and C. J. Taylor. Constrained active appearance models. In *Proc IEEE ICCV*, volume 1, pages 748–754, 2001.

[40] T. F. Cootes and C. J. Taylor. On representing edge structure for model matching. In *Proc IEEE CVPR*, volume 1, pages 1114–1119, 2001.

[41] T. F. Cootes and C. J. Taylor. Statistical models of appearance for computer vision. Technical report, University of Manchester, Wolfson Image Analysis Unit, Imaging Science and Biomedical Engineering, Manchester M13 9PT, United Kingdom, 2004.

[42] T. F. Cootes, C. J. Taylor, D. Cooper, and J. Graham. Training models of shape from sets of examples. In *Proc British Machine Vision Conference*, pages 9–18. Springer, 1992.

[43] T. F. Cootes, C. J. Taylor, D. H. Cooper, and J. Graham. Active shape models – their training and application. *Comput Vis Image Underst*, 61(1):38–59, 1995.

[44] T. F. Cootes, C. J. Taylor, and A. Lanitis. Active shape models: Evaluation of a multi-resolution method for improving search. In *Proc British Machine Vision Conference*, pages 327–336. BMVA Press, 1994.

[45] T. F. Cootes, C. Twining, V. Petrović, R. Schestowitz, and C. Taylor. Groupwise construction of appearance models using piece-wise affine deformations. In *Proc British Machine Vision Conference*, volume 2, pages 879–888, 2005.

[46] D. Cremers, M. Rousson, and R. Deriche. A review of statistical approaches to level set segmentation: Integrating color, texture, motion and shape. *Int J Comput Vis*, 72(2):195–215, 2007.

[47] D. Cristinacce and T. F. Cootes. Feature detection and tracking with constrained local models. In *Proc British Machine Vision Conference*, pages 929–938. BMVA Press, 2006.

[48] J. G. Csernansky, M. K. Schindler, N. R. Splinter, L. Wang, M. Gado, L. D. Selemon, D. Rastogi-Cruz, J. A. Posener, P. A. Thompson, and M. I. Miller. Abnormalities of thalamic volume and shape in schizophrenia. *Am J Psychiatry*, 161(5):896–902, May 2004.

[49] J. G. Daugman. Complete discrete 2-D Gabor transform by neural networks for image analysis and compression. *IEEE Trans on Acoustics, Speech and Signal Processing*, 36(7):1169–1179, Jul 1988.

[50] C. Davatzikos, D. Liu, D. Shen, and E. H. Herskovits. Spatial normalization of spine MR images for statistical correlation of lesions with clinical symptoms. *Radiology*, 224(3):919–926, Sep 2002.

[51] C. Davatzikos, X. Tao, and D. Shen. Hierarchical active shape models, using the wavelet transform. *IEEE Trans Med Imaging*, 22(3):414–423, Mar 2003.

[52] R. H. Davies. *Learning Shape: Optimal Models for Analysing Shape Variability*. PhD thesis, University of Manchester, 2002.

[53] R. H. Davies, C. J. Twining, P. D. Allen, T. F. Cootes, and C. J. Taylor. Building optimal 2D statistical shape models. *Image Vision Comput*, 21:1171–1182, Apr. 2003.

[54] R. H. Davies, C. J. Twining, P. D. Allen, T. F. Cootes, and C. J. Taylor. Shape discrimination in the hippocampus using an mdl model. In *Proc IPMI*, volume 2732 of *LNCS*, pages 38–50. Springer, Jul 2003.

[55] R. H. Davies, C. J. Twining, T. F. Cootes, J. C. Waterton, and C. J. Taylor. 3D statistical shape models using direct optimisation of description length. In *Proc ECCV*, volume 2352 of *LNCS*, pages 3–20. Springer, May 2002.

[56] R. H. Davies, C. J. Twining, T. F. Cootes, J. C. Waterton, and C. J. Taylor. A minimum description length approach to statistical shape modeling. *IEEE Trans Med Imaging*, 21(5):525–537, May 2002.

[57] M. de Bruijne, M. T. Lund, L. B. Tanko, P. P. Pettersen, and M. Nielsen. Quantitative vertebral morphometry using neighbor-conditional shape models. In *Proc MICCAI*, volume I, pages 1–8, 2006.

[58] M. de Bruijne and M. Nielsen. Shape particle filtering for image segmentation. In *Proc MICCAI*, volume 3216 of *LNCS*, pages 168–175. Springer, 2004.

[59] M. de Bruijne and M. Nielsen. Multi-object segmentation using shape particles. In *Proc IPMI*, volume 3565 of *LNCS*, pages 762–773. Springer, 2005.

[60] M. de Bruijne, B. van Ginneken, W. Niessen, J. Maintz, and M. Viergever. Active shape model based segmentation of abdominal

aortic aneurysms in CTA images. In M. Sonka and M. Fitzpatrick, editors, *Medical Imaging: Image Processing*, volume 4684 of *Proceedings of SPIE*, pages 463–474. SPIE Press, 2002.

[61] M. de Bruijne, B. van Ginneken, M. A. Viergever, and W. J. Niessen. Adapting active shape models for 3D segmentation of tubular structures in medical images. In *Proc IPMI*, volume 2732 of *LNCS*, pages 136–147. Springer, Jul 2003.

[62] M. de Bruijne, B. van Ginneken, M. A. Viergever, and W. J. Niessen. Interactive segmentation of abdominal aortic aneurysms in CTA images. *Med Image Anal*, 8(2):127–138, Jun 2004.

[63] F. De la Torre and M. J. Black. A framework for robust subspace learning. *Int J Comp Vis*, 54(1–3):117–142, 2003.

[64] F. Deligianni, A. J. Chung, and G.-Z. Yang. Nonrigid 2-D/3-D registration for patient specific bronchoscopy simulation with statistical shape modeling: phantom validation. *IEEE Trans Med Imaging*, 25(11):1462–1471, Nov 2006.

[65] H. Delingette. Simplex meshes: a general representation for 3D shape reconstruction. Technical Report 2214, INRIA, Sophia-Antipolis, France, 1994.

[66] A. P. Dempster, N. M. Laird, and D. B. Rubin. Maximum likelihood from incomplete data via the EM algorithm. *Journal of the Royal Statistical Society*, 39(1):1–38, 1977.

[67] M. Dickens, S. Gleason, and H. Sari-Sarraf. Volumetric segmentation via 3D active shape models. In *Proc IEEE Southwest Symposium on Image Analysis and Interpretation*, pages 248–252, 7-9 April 2002.

[68] R. Donner, M. Reiter, G. Langs, P. Peloschek, and H. Bischof. Fast active appearance model search using canonical correlation analysis. *IEEE Trans Pattern Anal Mach Intell*, 28(10):1690–1694, Oct. 2006.

[69] I. L. Dryden and K. V. Mardia. *Statistical shape analysis*. Wiley & Sons, 1998.

[70] S. Duchesne, J. Prussner, and D. L. Collins. Appearance-based segmentation of medial temporal lobe structures. *NeuroImage*, 17:515–531, 2002.

[71] N. Duta and M. Sonka. Segmentation and interpretation of MR brain images: an improved active shape model. *IEEE Trans Med Imaging*, 17(6):1049–1062, Dec 1998.

[72] A. Ericsson and K. Åström. Minimizing the description length using steepest descent. In *Proc British Machine Vision Conference*, pages 93–102, 2003.

[73] A. Ericsson and J. Karlsson. Aligning shapes by minimising the description length. In *Proc Scandinavian Conference on Image Analysis*, pages 709–718, 2005.

[74] A. Ericsson and J. Karlsson. Benchmarking of algorithms for automatic correspondence localisation. In *Proc British Machine Vision Conference*, pages 759–768. BMVA Press, 2006.

[75] L. Ferrarini, H. Olofsen, W. M. Palm, M. A. van Buchem, J. H. C. Reiber, and F. Admiraal-Behloul. GAMEs: Growing and adaptive meshes for fully automatic shape modeling and analysis. *Med Image Anal*, 11(3):302–314, Jun 2007.

[76] M. Fleute, S. Lavallée, and L. Desbat. Integrated approach for matching statistical shape models with intra-operative 2D and 3D data. In *Proc MICCAI*, volume 2489 of *LNCS*, pages 364–372. Springer, 2002.

[77] M. Fleute, S. Lavallée, and R. Julliard. Incorporating a statistically based shape model into a system for computer-assisted anterior cruciate ligament surgery. *Med Image Anal*, 3(3):209–222, Sep 1999.

[78] M. S. Floater and K. Hormann. *Tutorials on Multiresolution in Geometric Modelling*, chapter Parameterization of Triangulations and Unorganized Points, pages 287–316. Springer, 2002.

[79] M. S. Floater and K. Hormann. *Advances in Multiresolution for Geometric Modelling*, chapter Surface Parameterization: a Tutorial and Survey, pages 157–186. Springer, 2005.

[80] L. Florack, B. T. H. Romeny, M. Viergever, and J. Koenderink. The gaussian scale-space paradigm and the multiscale local jet. *Int J Comp Vis*, 18(1):61–75, 1996.

[81] L. J. Fogel, A. J. Owens, and M. J. Walsh. *Artificial Intelligence through Simulated Evolution*. John Wiley, New York, 1966.

[82] A. F. Frangi, D. Rueckert, J. A. Schnabel, and W. J. Niessen. Automatic 3D ASM construction via atlas-based landmarking and volumetric elastic registration. In *Proc IPMI*, volume 2082 of *LNCS*, pages 78–91. Springer, 2001.

[83] A. F. Frangi, D. Rueckert, J. A. Schnabel, and W. J. Niessen. Automatic construction of multiple-object three-dimensional statistical shape models: application to cardiac modeling. *IEEE Trans Med Imaging*, 21(9):1151–1166, Sep 2002.

[84] D. Freedman, R. Radke, T. Zhang, Y. Jeong, D. Lovelock, and G. Chen. Model-based segmentation of medical imagery by matching distributions. *IEEE Trans Med Imaging*, 24(3):281–292, March 2005.

[85] W. T. Freeman and E. H. Adelson. The design and use of steerable filters. *IEEE Trans Pattern Anal Mach Intell*, 13(9):891–906, Sep 1991.

[86] Y. Freund and R. Schapire. A decision-theoretic generalization of on-line learning and an application to boosting. *J Computer and System Sciences*, 55(1):119–139, Aug 1997.

[87] J. Fripp, S. Crozier, S. Warfield, and S. Ourselin. Automatic initialization of 3D deformable models for cartilage segmentation. In *Proc Digital Image Computing: Techniques and Applications*, pages 513–518, Dec. 2005.

[88] J. Fripp, S. Crozier, S. K. Warfield, and S. Ourselin. Automatic segmentation of the knee bones using 3D active shape models. In *Proc ICPR*, volume 1, pages 167–170, August 2006.

[89] D. Fritz, D. Rinck, R. Dillmann, and M. Scheuering. Segmentation of the left and right cardiac ventricle using a combined bi-temporal statistical model. In K. R. Cleary and R. L. Galloway, editors, *Proc SPIE Medical Imaging: Visualization, Image-guided Procedures, and Display*, volume 6141, pages 605–614, San Diego, CA, 2006. SPIE Press.

[90] D. Fritz, D. Rinck, R. Unterhinninghofen, R. Dillmann, and M. Scheuering. Automatic segmentation of the left ventricle and computation of diagnostic parameters using regiongrowing and a statistical model. In J. M. Fitzpatrick and J. M. Reinhardt, editors, *Proc SPIE Medical Imaging: Image Processing*, volume 5747, pages 1844–1854, San Diego, CA, 2005. SPIE Press.

[91] G. Gerig, M. Jomier, and M. Chakos. Valmet: a new validation tool for assessing and improving 3D object segmentation. In *Proc MICCAI*, volume 2208 of *LNCS*, pages 516–523. Springer, 2001.

[92] S. Gold, A. Rangarajan, C.-P. Lu, S. Pappu, and E. Mjolsness. New algorithms for 2D and 3D point matching: Pose estimation and correspondence. *Pattern Recognition*, 31:1019–1031, 1998.

[93] P. Golland, W. E. L. Grimson, M. E. Shenton, and R. Kikinis. Detection and analysis of statistical differences in anatomical shape. *Med Image Anal*, 9(1):69–86, Feb 2005.

[94] C. Goodall. Procrustes methods in the statistical analysis of shape. *J Roy Stat Soc B*, 53(2):285–339, 1991.

[95] J. C. Gower. Generalized Procrustes analysis. *Psychometrika*, 40:33–51, 1975.

[96] X. Gu, Y. Wang, T. F. Chan, P. M. Thompson, and S. T. Yau. Genus zero surface conformal mapping and its application to brain surface mapping. In *Proc. IPMI*, pages 172–184, 2003.

[97] H. Handels, A. Horsch, and H.-P. Meinzer. Andvances in medical image computing. *Methods Inf Med*, 46(3):251–253, 2007.

[98] J. Haslam, C. J. Taylor, and T. F. Cootes. A probabilistic fitness measure for deformable template models. In *Proc British Machine Vision Conference*, pages 33–42. BMVA Press, 1994.

[99] D. J. Hawkes, D. Barratt, J. M. Blackall, C. Chan, P. J. Edwards, K. Rhode, G. P. Penney, J. McClelland, and D. L. G. Hill. Tissue deformation and shape models in image-guided interventions: a discussion paper. *Med Image Anal*, 9(2):163–175, Apr 2005.

[100] T. Heimann, S. Münzing, H.-P. Meinzer, and I. Wolf. A shape-guided deformable model with evolutionary algorithm initialization for 3D soft tissue segmentation. In *Proc IPMI*, volume 4584 of *LNCS*, pages 1–12. Springer, 2007.

[101] T. Heimann, I. Oguz, I. Wolf, M. Styner, and H.-P. Meinzer. Implementing the automatic generation of 3D statistical shape models with ITK. In *Proc MICCAI Open Science Workshop*, 2006.

[102] T. Heimann, I. Wolf, and H.-P. Meinzer. Automatic generation of 3D statistical shape models with optimal landmark distributions. *Methods Inf Med*, 46(3):275–281, 2007.

[103] T. Heimann, I. Wolf, T. G. Williams, and H.-P. Meinzer. 3D Active Shape Models using gradient descent optimization of description length. In *Proc IPMI*, volume 3565 of *LNCS*, pages 566–577. Springer, 2005.

[104] P. Heinze, D. Meister, R. Kober, J. Raczkowsky, and H. Wörn. Atlas-based segmentation of pathological knee joints. *Stud Health Technol Inform*, 85:198–203, 2002.

[105] G. Heitz, T. Rohlfing, and C. R. Maurer. Automatic generation of shape models using nonrigid registration with a single segmented template mesh. In *Proc Int Workshop on Vision, Modeling, and Visualization*, pages 73–80, November 2004.

[106] G. Heitz, T. Rohlfing, and C. R. Maurer. Statistical shape model generation using nonrigid deformation of a template mesh. In J. M. Fitzpatrick and J. M. Reinhardt, editors, *Proc SPIE Medical Imaging: Image Processing*, volume 5747, pages 1411–1421, San Diego, CA, 2005. SPIE Press.

[107] K. B. Hilger, R. Larsen, and M. C. Wrobel. Growth modeling of human mandibles using non-euclidean metrics. *Med Image Anal*, 7(4):425–433, Dec 2003.

[108] A. Hill, T. F. Cootes, and C. J. Taylor. A generic system for image interpretation using flexible templates. In *Proc British Machine Vision Conference*, pages 276–285, Leeds, England, Sep 1992.

[109] A. Hill, T. F. Cootes, and C. J. Taylor. Active shape models and the shape approximation problem. *Image Vision Comput*, 14(8):601–607, August 1996.

[110] A. Hill and C. J. Taylor. Model-based image interpretation using genetic algorithms. *Image Vision Comput*, 10(5):295–300, 1992.

[111] A. Hill, C. J. Taylor, and A. D. Brett. A framework for automatic landmark identification using a new method of nonrigid correspondence. *IEEE Trans Pattern Anal Mach Intell*, 22(3):241–251, March 2000.

[112] S. Ho and G. Gerig. Profile scale-spaces for multiscale image match. In *Proc MICCAI*, volume 3216 of *LNCS*, pages 176–183. Springer, 2004.

[113] A. C. Hodge, A. Fenster, D. B. Downey, and H. M. Ladak. Prostate boundary segmentation from ultrasound images using 2D active shape models: Optimisation and extension to 3D. *Comput Methods Programs Biomed*, 84(2-3):99–113, Dec 2006.

[114] J. H. Holland. *Adaption in Natural and Artificial Systems*. University of Michigan Press, 1975.

[115] P. Horkaew and G. Z. Yang. Optimal deformable surface models for 3D medical image analysis. In *Proc IPMI*, volume 2732 of *LNCS*, pages 13–24. Springer, Jul 2003.

[116] X. Hou, S. Li, H. Zhang, and Q. Cheng. Direct appearance models. In *Proc IEEE CVPR*, volume 1, pages 828–833, 2001.

[117] J. Hug, C. Brechbühler, and G. Székely. Model-based initialisation for segmentation. In *Proc ECCV*, pages 290–306, 2000.

[118] T. J. Hutton, B. F. Buxton, and P. Hammond. Dense surface point distribution models of the human face. In L. Staib, editor, *IEEE Workshop on Mathematical Methods in Biomedical Image Analysis*, pages 153–160, 2001.

[119] A. Hyvärinen, J. Karhunen, and E. Oja. *Independent Component Analysis*. John Wiley & Sons, 2001.

[120] M. Isard and A. Blake. Condensation – conditional density propagation for visual tracking. *Int J Comp Vis*, 29(1):5–28, 1998.

[121] A. K. Jain, Y. Zhong, and M.-P. Dubuisson-Jolly. Deformable template models: a review. *Signal Process*, 71(2):109–129, 1998.

[122] F. Jiao, S. Li, H.-Y. Shum, and D. Schuurmans. Face alignment using statistical models and wavelet features. In *Proc IEEE CVPR*, volume 1, pages 321–327, Jun 2003.

[123] K. Josephson, A. Ericsson, and J. Karlsson. Segmentation of medical images using three-dimensional active shape models. In *Proc Scandinavian Conference on Image Analysis*, volume 3540 of *LNCS*, pages 719–728. Springer, 2005.

[124] D. Kalman. A singularly valuable decomposition: the SVD of a matrix. *College Math Journal*, 27:2–23, 1996.

[125] M. Kass, A. Witkin, and D. Terzopoulos. Snakes: Active contour models. *Int J Comp Vis*, 1(4):321–331, 1988.

[126] M. R. Kaus, V. Pekar, C. Lorenz, R. Truyen, S. Lobregt, and J. Weese. Automated 3-D PDM construction from segmented images using deformable models. *IEEE Trans Med Imaging*, 22(8):1005–1013, Aug 2003.

[127] M. R. Kaus, J. von Berg, J. Weese, W. Niessen, and V. Pekar. Automated segmentation of the left ventricle in cardiac MRI. *Med Image Anal*, 8(3):245–254, Sep 2004.

[128] A. Kelemen, G. Székely, and G. Gerig. Elastic model-based segmentation of 3-D neuroradiological data sets. *IEEE Trans Med Imaging*, 18(10):828–839, Oct 1999.

[129] D. G. Kendall. A survey of the statistical theory of shape. *Statistical Science*, 4(2):87–120, 1989.

[130] S. H. Kim, J.-M. Lee, H.-P. Kim, D. P. Jang, Y.-W. Shin, T. H. Ha, J.-J. Kim, I. Y. Kim, J. S. Kwon, and S. I. Kim. Asymmetry analysis of deformable hippocampal model using the principal component in schizophrenia. *Hum Brain Mapp*, 25(4):361–369, Aug 2005.

[131] J. Kittler and F. M. Alkoot. Moderating k-NN classifiers. *Pattern Analysis & Applications*, 5(3):326–332, 2002.

[132] J. Klemencic, J. P. W. Pluim, M. A. Viergever, H. G. Schnack, and V. Valencic. Non-rigid registration based active appearance models for 3D medical image segmentation. *J Imaging Sci Technol*, 48:166–171, 2004.

[133] S. Klim, S. Mortensen, B. Bodvarsson, L. Hyldstrup, and H. H. Thodberg. More active shape model. In *Proc Image and Vision Computing*, pages 396–401, New Zealand, Nov 2003.

[134] L. Kobbelt, S. Campagna, and H.-P. Seidel. A general framework for mesh decimation. In *Proc Graphics Interface*, pages 43–50, 1998.

[135] A. C. W. Kotcheff and C. J. Taylor. Automatic construction of eigen-shape models by direct optimization. *Med Image Anal*, 2(4):303–314, 1998.

[136] H. Lamecker, T. Lange, and M. Seebaß. A statistical shape model for the liver. In T. Dohi and R. Kikinis, editors, *Proc MICCAI*, volume 2489 of *LNCS*, pages 422–427. Springer, 2002.

[137] H. Lamecker, T. Lange, and M. Seebaß. Segmentation of the liver using a 3D statistical shape model. Technical report, Zuse Institute, Berlin, 2004.

[138] H. Lamecker, T. Lange, M. Seebaß, S. Eulenstein, M. Westerhoff, and H. C. Hege. Automatic segmentation of the liver for preoperative planning of resections. *Stud Health Technol Inform*, 94:171–173, 2003.

[139] H. Lamecker, M. Seebaß, H.-C. Hege, and P. Deuflhard. A 3D statistical shape model of the pelvic bone for segmentation. In J. M. Fitzpatrick and M. Sonka, editors, *Proc SPIE Medical Imaging: Image Processing*, volume 5370, pages 1341–1351, 2004.

[140] G. Langs, P. Peloschek, R. Donner, M. Reiter, and H. Bischof. Active feature models. In *Proc ICPR*, volume 1, pages 417–420, 20-24 Aug. 2006.

[141] Z. Lao, D. Shen, and C. Davatzikos. Statistical shape model for automatic skull-stripping of brain images. In *Proc IEEE Int Symposium on Biomedical Imaging*, pages 855–858, 7-10 July 2002.

[142] R. M. Lapp, M. Lorenzo-Valdés, and D. Rueckert. 3D/4D cardiac segmentation using active appearance models, non-rigid registration, and the Insight toolkit. In C. Barillot, D. R. Haynor, and P. Hellier, editors, *Proc MICCAI*, volume 3216 of *LNCS*, pages 419–426. Springer, 2004.

[143] R. Larsen and H. Eiriksson. Robust and resistant 2D shape alignment. Technical report, IMM at DTU, 2001.

[144] R. Larsen and K. B. Hilger. Statistical shape analysis using non-euclidean metrics. *Med Image Anal*, 7(4):417–423, Dec 2003.

[145] R. Larsen, M. B. Stegmann, S. Darkner, S. Forchhammer, T. F. Cootes, and B. K. Ersbøll. Texture enhanced appearance models. *Comp Vis Image Underst*, 106(1):20–30, Apr 2007.

[146] S.-L. Lee, P. Horkaew, W. Caspersz, A. Darzi, and G.-Z. Yang. Assessment of shape variation of the levator ani with optimal scan planning and statistical shape modeling. *J Comput Assist Tomogr*, 29(2):154–162, 2005.

[147] K. Lekadir, R. Merrifield, and G.-Z. Yang. Outlier detection and handling for robust 3-D active shape models search. *IEEE Trans Med Imaging*, 26(2):212–222, Feb 2007.

[148] M. E. Leventon, W. E. L. Grimson, and O. Faugeras. Statistical shape influence in geodesic active contours. In *Proc IEEE CVPR*, volume 1, pages 316–323, June 2000.

[149] B. Li and J. M. Reinhardt. Automatic generation of 3-D shape models and their application to tomographic image segmentation. In *Proc SPIE Medical Imaging*, volume 4322, pages 311–322, San Diego, CA, 17-22 Feb. 2001.

[150] H. Li and O. Chutatape. Automated feature extraction in color retinal images by a model based approach. *IEEE Trans Biomed Eng*, 51(2):246–254, Feb 2004.

[151] K. Li, S. Millington, X. Wu, D. Z. Chen, and M. Sonka. Simultaneous segmentation of multiple closed surfaces using optimal graph searching. In *Proc IPMI*, volume 3565 of *LNCS*, pages 406–417. Springer, 2005.

[152] S. Y. Li, L. T. Zhu, and T. Z. Jiang. Active shape model segmentation using local edge structures and AdaBoost. In *Proc Medical Imaging and Augmented Reality*, volume 3150 of *LNCS*, pages 121–128. Springer, 2004.

[153] Y. Li and W. Ito. Shape parameter optimization for adaboosted active shape model. In *Proc IEEE ICCV*, volume 1, pages 251–258, 17-21 Oct. 2005.

[154] Z. Li and H. Ai. Texture-constrained shape prediction for mouth contour extraction and its state estimation. In *Proc ICPR*, volume 2, pages 88–91, 20-24 Aug. 2006.

[155] S.-J. Lim and Y.-S. Ho. 3-D active shape image segmentation using a scale model. In *Proc IEEE Symposium on Signal Processing and Information Technology*, pages 168–173, 2006.

[156] W. E. Lorensen and H. E. Cline. Marching cubes: A high resolution 3D surface construction algorithm. In *SIGGRAPH '87: Proceedings of the 14th annual conference on Computer graphics and interactive techniques*, pages 163–169, New York, NY, USA, 1987. ACM Press.

[157] C. Lorenz and N. Krahnstöver. Generation of point-based 3D statistical shape models for anatomical objects. *Comput Vis Image Underst*, 77(2):175–191, 2000.

[158] C. Lorenz and J. von Berg. A comprehensive shape model of the heart. *Med Image Anal*, 10(4):657–670, Aug 2006.

[159] J. Lötjönen, K. Antila, E. Lamminmäki, J. Koikkalainen, M. Lilja, and T. F. Cootes. Artificial enlargement of a training set for statistical shape models: Application to cardiac images. In A. F. Frangi, P. Radeva, and A. S. ad M. Hernandez, editors, *Proc Functional Imaging and Modeling of the Heart*, volume 3504 of *LNCS*, pages 92–101. Springer, 2005.

[160] J. Lötjönen, S. Kivistö, J. Koikkalainen, D. Smutek, and K. Lauerma. Statistical shape model of atria, ventricles and epicardium from short- and long-axis MR images. *Med Image Anal*, 8(3):371–386, Sep 2004.

[161] R. Malladi, J. Sethian, and B. Vemuri. Shape modeling with front propagation: A level set approach. *IEEE Trans Pattern Anal Mach Intell*, pages 158–174, 1995.

[162] A. Matheny and D. B. Goldgof. The use of three- and four-dimensional surface harmonics for rigid and nonrigid shape recovery and representation. *IEEE Trans Pattern Anal Mach Intell*, 17(10):967–981, 1995.

[163] I. Matthews and S. Baker. Active appearance models revisited. *Int J Comp Vis*, 60:135–164, 2004.

[164] T. McInerney and D. Terzopoulos. Deformable models in medical image analysis: a survey. *Med Image Anal*, 1(2):91–108, Jun 1996.

[165] T. McInerney and D. Terzopoulos. Topology adaptive deformable surfaces for medical image volume segmentation. *IEEE Trans Med Imaging*, 18(10):840–850, Oct 1999.

[166] S. J. McKenna, S. Gong, R. P. Würtz, J. Tanner, and D. Banin. Tracking facial feature points with Gabor wavelets and shape models. In *Proc Int Conf on Audio- and Video-Based Biometric Person Authentication*, pages 35–42, London, UK, 1997. Springer.

[167] D. Meier and E. Fisher. Parameter space warping: shape-based correspondence between morphologically different objects. *IEEE Trans Med Imaging*, 21(1):31–47, Jan. 2002.

[168] H.-P. Meinzer, M. Thorn, and C. E. Cardenas. Computerized planning of liver surgery – an overview. *Computers & Graphics*, 26(4):569–576, 2002.

[169] S. Mitchell, J. Bosch, B. Lelieveldt, R. van der Geest, J. Reiber, and M. Sonka. 3-D active appearance models: segmentation of cardiac MR and ultrasound images. *IEEE Trans Med Imaging*, 21(9):1167–1178, Sept. 2002.

[170] T. Möller and B. Trumbore. Fast, minimum storage ray-triangle intersection. *Journal of Graphics Tools*, 2:21–28, 1997.

[171] J. Montagnat, H. Delingette, and N. Ayache. A review of deformable surfaces: topology, geometry and deformation. *Image Vision Comput*, 19(14):1023–1040, 2001.

[172] S. Muraki. Volume data and wavelet transforms. *IEEE Computer Graphics and Applications*, 13(4):50–56, Jul 1993.

[173] J. Nahed, M.-P. Jolly, and G.-Z. Yang. Robust active shape models: A robust, generic and simple automatic segmentation tool. In *Proc MICCAI*, volume 4191 of *LNCS*, pages 1–8. Springer, 2006.

[174] D. Nain, S. Haker, A. Bobick, and A. Tannenbaum. Multiscale 3-D shape representation and segmentation using spherical wavelets. *IEEE Trans Med Imaging*, 26(4):598–618, April 2007.

[175] A. Neumann and C. Lorenz. Statistical shape model based segmentation of medical images. *Comput Med Imag Grap*, 22(2):133–143, 1998.

[176] W. J. Niessen, C. J. Bouma, K. L. Vincken, and M. A. Viergever. *Performance Characterization in Computer Vision*, chapter Error metrics for quantitative evaluation of medical image segmentation, pages 275–284. Kluwer Academic, 2000.

[177] C. Nikou, G. Bueno, F. Heitz, and J. P. Armspach. A joint physics-based statistical deformable model for multimodal brain image analysis. *IEEE Trans Med Imaging*, 20(10):1026–1037, Oct 2001.

[178] S. Ordás, L. Boisrobert, M. Bossa, M. Huguet, M. Laucelli, S. Olmos, and A. Frangi. Grid-enabled automatic construction of a two-chamber cardiac PDM from a large database of dynamic 3D shapes. In *Proc IEEE Int Symposium on Biomedical Imaging*, pages 416–419, 2004.

[179] S. Ordás, L. Boisrobert, M. Huguet, and A. Frangi. Active shape models with invariant optimal features (IOF-ASM) application to cardiac MRI segmentation. In *Proc Computers in Cardiology*, pages 633–636, 21-24 Sept. 2003.

[180] S. Osher and J. A. Sethian. Fronts propagating with curvature-dependent speed: Algorithms based on Hamilton-Jacobi formulation. *J Comput Phys*, 79:12–49, 1988.

[181] V. Ostromoukhov. A simple and efficient error-diffusion algorithm. In *Proc. SIGGRAPH*, pages 567–572. ACM Press, 2001.

[182] T. Papadopoulo and M. I. A. Lourakis. Estimating the jacobian of the singular value decomposition: theory and applications. In *Proc. ECCV*, pages 554–570, 2000.

[183] H. Park, P. Bland, and C. Meyer. Construction of an abdominal probabilistic atlas and its application in segmentation. *IEEE Trans Med Imaging*, 22(4):483–492, April 2003.

[184] R. Paulsen, R. Larsen, C. Nielsen, S. Laugesen, and B. K. Ersboll. Building and testing a statistical shape model of the human ear canal. In *Proc MICCAI*, volume 2489 of *LNCS*, pages 373–380. Springer, 2002.

[185] R. R. Paulsen and K. B. Hilger. Shape modelling using markov random field restoration of point correspondences. In *Proc IPMI*, volume 2732 of *LNCS*, pages 1–12. Springer, Jul 2003.

[186] V. Pekar, M. R. Kaus, C. Lorenz, S. Lobregt, R. Truyen, and J. Weese. Shape-model-based adaptation of 3D deformable meshes for segmentation of medical images. In M. Sonka and K. M. Hanson, editors, *Proc SPIE Medical Imaging: Image Processing*, volume 4322, pages 281–289, San Diego, CA, 2001.

[187] V. Pekar, T. R. McNutt, and M. R. Kaus. Automated model-based organ delineation for radiotherapy planning in prostatic region. *Int J Radiat Oncol Biol Phys*, 60(3):973–980, Nov 2004.

[188] P. Perona and J. Malik. Scale-space and edge detection using anisotropic diffusion. *IEEE Trans Pattern Anal Mach Intell*, 12(7):629–639, Jul 1990.

[189] J. Peters, O. Ecabert, and J. Weese. Feature optimization via simulated search for model-based heart segmentation. In *Proc Computer Assisted Radiology and Surgery*, pages 33–38. Elsevier, 2005.

[190] G. Peyre and L. D. Cohen. Geodesic re-meshing and parameterization using front propagation. In *Proc. IEEE Workshop on Variational and Level Set Methods*, pages 33–40, 2003.

[191] A. Pitiot, H. Delingette, and P. M. Thompson. Learning shape correspondence for n-D curves. *Int J Comp Vis*, 71(1):71–88, January 2007.

[192] A. Pitiot, A. W. Toga, and P. M. Thompson. Adaptive elastic segmentation of brain MRI via shape-model-guided evolutionary programming. *IEEE Trans Med Imaging*, 21(8):910–923, Aug 2002.

[193] S. M. Pizer, P. T. Fletcher, Y. Fridman, D. S. Fritsch, A. G. Gash, J. M. Glotzer, S. Joshi, A. Thall, J. Z. Chen, and et al. Deformable m-reps for 3D medical image segmentation. *Int J Comp Vis*, 55(2/3):85–106, 2003.

[194] S. M. Pizer, D. S. Fritsch, P. A. Yushkevich, V. E. Johnson, and E. L. Chaney. Segmentation, registration, and measurement of shape variation via image object shape. *IEEE Trans Med Imaging*, 18(10):851–865, October 1999.

[195] S. M. Pizer, J.-Y. Jeong, C. Lu, K. Muller, and S. Joshi. Estimating the statistics of multi-object anatomic geometry using inter-object

relationships. In *Proc. Deep Structure, Singularities, and Computer Vision*, volume 3753 of *LNCS*, pages 60–71. Springer, 2005.

[196] C. Plathow, M. Schoebinger, C. Fink, S. Ley, M. Puderbach, M. Eichinger, M. Bock, H.-P. Meinzer, and H.-U. Kauczor. Evaluation of lung volumetry using dynamic three-dimensional magnetic resonance imaging. *Invest Radiol*, 40(3):173–179, Mar 2005.

[197] K. M. Pohl, J. Fisher, M. Shenton, R. W. McCarley, W. E. L. Grimson, R. Kikinis, and W. M. Wells. Logarithm odds maps for shape representation. In *Proc MICCAI*, volume 4191 of *LNCS*, pages 955–963. Springer, October 2006.

[198] E. Praun, W. Sweldens, and P. Schröder. Consistent mesh parameterizations. In *Proc SIGGRAPH*, pages 179–184, 2001.

[199] K. T. Rajamani, M. A. Styner, H. Talib, G. Zheng, L. P. Nolte, and M. A. G. Ballester. Statistical deformable bone models for robust 3D surface extrapolation from sparse data. *Med Image Anal*, 11(2):99–109, Apr 2007.

[200] A. Rangarajan, H. Chui, and F. L. Bookstein. The softassign procrustes matching algorithm. In *Proc IPMI*, volume 1230 of *LNCS*, pages 29–42. Springer, 1997.

[201] M. Rao, J. Stough, Y.-Y. Chi, K. Muller, G. Tracton, S. M. Pizer, and E. L. Chaney. Comparison of human and automatic segmentations of kidneys from CT images. *Int J Radiat Oncol Biol Phys*, 61(3):954–960, Mar 2005.

[202] M. Roberts, T. F. Cootes, and J. Adams. Vertebral shape: automatic measurement with dynamically sequenced active appearance models. In *Proc MICCAI*, volume 3750 of *LNCS*, pages 733–740. Springer, 2005.

[203] M. Rogers and J. Graham. Robust active shape model search. In *Proc ECCV*, pages 517–530. Springer, 2002.

[204] D. Rueckert, A. Frangi, and J. Schnabel. Automatic construction of 3-D statistical deformation models of the brain using nonrigid registration. *IEEE Trans Med Imaging*, 22(8):1014–1025, 2003.

[205] H.-P. Schwefel. *Evolution and Optimum Seeking.* John Wiley & Sons, Inc., New York, 1995.

[206] I. M. Scott, T. F. Cootes, and C. J. Taylor. Improving appearance model matching using local image structure. In *Proc IPMI*, volume 2732 of *LNCS*, pages 258–269. Springer, 2003.

[207] Y. Shang and O. Dossel. Statistical 3D shape-model guided segmentation of cardiac images. In *Proc Computers in Cardiology*, pages 553–556, 19-22 Sept. 2004.

[208] C. Shannon. A mathematical theory of communication. *Bell System Technical Journal*, 27:379–423, 623–656, 1948.

[209] C. R. Shelton. Morphable surface models. *Int J Comp Vis*, 38(1):75–91, 2000.

[210] D. Shen, E. H. Herskovits, and C. Davatzikos. An adaptive-focus statistical shape model for segmentation and shape modeling of 3-D brain structures. *IEEE Trans Med Imaging*, 20(4):257–270, Apr 2001.

[211] D. Shen, S. Moffat, S. M. Resnick, and C. Davatzikos. Measuring size and shape of the hippocampus in MR images using a deformable shape model. *Neuroimage*, 15(2):422–434, Feb 2002.

[212] D. Shen, Y. Zhan, and C. Davatzikos. Segmentation of prostate boundaries from ultrasound images using statistical shape model. *IEEE Trans Med Imaging*, 22(4):539–551, Apr 2003.

[213] M. E. Shenton, G. Gerig, R. W. McCarley, G. Székely, and R. Kikinis. Amygdala-hippocampal shape differences in schizophrenia: the application of 3D shape models to volumetric MR data. *Psychiatry Res.*, 115(1–2)(1):15–35, 2002.

[214] R. Sierra, G. Zsemlye, G. Székely, and M. Bajka. Generation of variable anatomical models for surgical training simulators. *Med Image Anal*, 10(2):275–285, Apr 2006.

[215] K. Sjöstrand, M. B. Stegmann, and R. Larsen. Sparse principal component analysis in medical shape modeling. In *Proc SPIE Medical Imaging: Image Processing*, volume 6144, pages 1579–1590. SPIE Press, feb 2006.

[216] L. Soler, H. Delingette, G. Malandain, J. Montagnat, N. Ayache, C. Koehl, O. Dourthe, B. Malassagne, M. Smith, D. Mutter, and J. Marescaux. Fully automatic anatomical, pathological, and functional segmentation from ct scans for hepatic surgery. *Comput Aided Surg*, 6(3):131–142, 2001.

[217] P. D. Sozou, T. F. Cootes, C. J. Taylor, and E. C. Di-Mauro. A nonlinear generalisation of PDMs using polynomial regression. In *Proc British Machine Vision Conference*, pages 397–406, Surrey, UK, 1994. BMVA Press.

[218] P. D. Sozou, T. F. Cootes, C. J. Taylor, and E. C. D. Mauro. Non-linear point distribution modelling using a multi-layer perceptron. In *Proc British Machine Vision Conference*, pages 107–116, Surrey, UK, 1995. BMVA Press.

[219] L. H. Staib and J. S. Duncan. Model-based deformable surface finding for medical images. *IEEE Trans Med Imaging*, 15(5):720–731, Oct. 1996.

[220] M. B. Stegmann, B. K. Ersboll, and R. Larsen. FAME – a flexible appearance modeling environment. *IEEE Trans Med Imaging*, 22(10):1319–1331, Oct. 2003.

[221] M. B. Stegmann, R. Fisker, and B. K. Ersbøll. Extending and applying active appearance models for automated, high precision segmentation in different image modalities. In I. Austvoll, editor, *Proc Scandinavian Conference on Image Analysis*, pages 90–97, Stavanger, Norway, jun 2001. NOBIM.

[222] M. B. Stegmann and R. Larsen. Multi-band modelling of appearance. *Image and Vision Computing*, 21(1):61–67, jan 2003.

[223] M. B. Stegmann and D. Pedersen. Bi-temporal 3D active appearance models with applications to unsupervised ejection fraction estimation. In J. M. Fitzpatrick and J. M. Reinhardt, editors, *Proc SPIE Medical Imaging*, volume 5747, pages 336–350, San Diego, CA, Feb 2005. SPIE Press.

[224] M. B. Stegmann, K. Sjöstrand, and R. Larsen. Sparse modeling of landmark and texture variability using the orthomax criterion. In

*Proc SPIE Medical Imaging: Image Processing*, volume 6144, pages 485–496. SPIE Press, feb 2006.

[225] J. Stough, P. M. Pizer, E. L. Chaney, and M. Rao. Clustering on image boundary regions for deformable model segmentation. In *Proc IEEE Int Symposium on Biomedical Imaging*, volume 1, pages 436–43, 2004.

[226] M. A. Styner, G. Gerig, J. Lieberman, D. Jones, and D. Weinberger. Statistical shape analysis of neuroanatomical structures based on medial models. *Med Image Anal*, 7(3):207–220, Sep 2003.

[227] M. A. Styner, J. A. Lieberman, D. Pantazis, and G. Gerig. Boundary and medial shape analysis of the hippocampus in schizophrenia. *Med Image Anal*, 8(3):197–203, Sep 2004.

[228] M. A. Styner, K. T. Rajamani, L.-P. Nolte, G. Zsemlye, G. Székely, C. J. Taylor, and R. H. Davies. Evaluation of 3D correspondence methods for model building. In *Proc IPMI*, volume 2732 of *LNCS*, pages 63–75. Springer, Jul 2003.

[229] M. A. Styner, S. Xu, M. El-Sayed, and G. Gerig. Correspondence evaluation in local shape analysis and structural subdivision. In *Proc IEEE Int Symposium on Biomedical Imaging*, pages 1192–1195, April 2007.

[230] G. Subsol, J.-P. Thirion, and N. Ayache. A scheme for automatically building three-dimensional morphometric anatomical atlases: application to a skull atlas. *Med Image Anal*, 2(1):37–60, 1998.

[231] A. Suinesiaputra, A. F. Frangi, M. Üzümcü, J. H. C. Reiber, and B. P. F. Lelieveldt. Extraction of myocardial contractility patterns from short-axes MR images using independent component analysis. In M. Sonka, I. Kakadiaris, and J. Kybic, editors, *Proc IEEE Workshop on Mathematical Methods in Biomedical Image Analysis*, volume 3117 of *LNCS*, pages 75–86. Springer, 2004.

[232] V. Surazhsky and C. Gotsman. Explicit surface remeshing. In *Proc. Eurographics Symposium on Geometry Processing*, pages 17–28, Aachen, Germany, 2003.

[233] G. Székely, A. Kelemen, C. Brechbühler, and G. Gerig. Segmentation of 2-D and 3-D objects from MRI volume data using constrained elastic deformations of flexible Fourier contour and surface models. *Med Image Anal*, 1(1):19–34, Mar 1996.

[234] R. Szeliski and S. Lavallée. Matching 3-D anatomical surfaces with non-rigid deformations using octree-splines. *Int J Comp Vis*, 18(2):171–186, 1996.

[235] T. S. Y. Tang and R. E. Ellis. 2D/3D deformable registration using a hybrid atlas. In *Proc MICCAI*, volume 3750 of *LNCS*, pages 223–230. Springer, 2005.

[236] T. T. Tanimoto. An elementary mathematical theory of classification and prediction. Technical report, IBM Research, 1958.

[237] X. Tao, J. L. Prince, and C. Davatzikos. Using a statistical shape model to extract sulcal curves on the outer cortex of the human brain. *IEEE Trans Med Imaging*, 21(5):513–524, May 2002.

[238] D. Terzopoulos, A. Witkin, and M. Kass. Constraints on deformable models: recovering 3D shape and nongrid motion. *Artif Intell*, 36(1):91–123, 1988.

[239] H. H. Thodberg. Minimum description length shape and appearance models. In *Proc IPMI*, volume 2732 of *LNCS*, pages 51–62. Springer, July 2003.

[240] H. H. Thodberg and H. Olafsdottir. Adding curvature to minimum description length shape models. In *Proc British Machine Vision Conference*, pages 251–260. BMVA Press, 2003.

[241] P. M. Thompson, K. M. Hayashi, G. I. D. Zubicaray, A. L. Janke, S. E. Rose, J. Semple, M. S. Hong, D. H. Herman, D. Gravano, D. M. Doddrell, and A. W. Toga. Mapping hippocampal and ventricular change in alzheimer disease. *Neuroimage*, 22(4):1754–1766, Aug 2004.

[242] P. M. Thompson, C. Schwartz, and A. W. Toga. High-resolution random mesh algorithms for creating a probabilistic 3D surface atlas of the human brain. *Neuroimage*, 3(1):19–34, Feb 1996.

[243] P. M. Thompson and A. W. Toga. Detection, visualization and animation of abnormal anatomic structure with a deformable probabilistic brain atlas based on random vector field transformations. *Med Image Anal*, 1(4):271–294, 1997.

[244] T. Tölli, J. Koikkalainen, K. Lauerma, and J. Lötjönen. Artificially enlarged training set in image segmentation. In *Proc MICCAI*, volume 4190 of *LNCS*, pages 75–82. Springer, 2006.

[245] B. Tsagaan, A. Shimizu, H. Kobatake, and K. Miyakawa. An automated segmentation method of kidney using statistical information. In *Proc MICCAI*, volume 2488 of *LNCS*, pages 556–563. Springer, 2002.

[246] A. Tsai, J. Yezzi, A., W. Wells, C. Tempany, D. Tucker, A. Fan, W. Grimson, and A. Willsky. A shape-based approach to the segmentation of medical imagery using level sets. *IEEE Trans Med Imaging*, 22(2):137–154, Feb. 2003.

[247] C. J. Twining, T. F. Cootes, S. Marsland, V. Petrovic, R. Schestowitz, and C. J. Taylor. A unified information-theoretic approach to groupwise non-rigid registration and model building. In G. E. Christensen and M. Sonka, editors, *Proc IPMI*, volume 3565 of *LNCS*, pages 1–14. Springer, 2005.

[248] C. J. Twining and C. J. Taylor. Kernel principal component analysis and the construction of non-linear active shape models. In *Proc British Machine Vision Conference*, pages 23–32. BMVA Press, 2001.

[249] M. Üzümcü, A. F. Frangi, J. H. C. Reiber, and B. P. F. Lelieveldt. Independent component analysis in statistical shape models. In *Proc SPIE Medical Imaging*, volume 5032, pages 375–383, 2003.

[250] H. C. van Assen. *3D Active Shape Modeling for cardiac MR and CT image segmentation*, chapter Assessment of an autolandmarked statistical shape model, pages 71–82. Number ISBN 90-8559-163-5. Optima Grafische Communicatie, Rotterdam, 2006.

[251] H. C. van Assen, M. G. Danilouchkine, F. Behloul, H. J. Lamb, R. J. van der Geest, J. H. C. Reiber, and B. P. F. Lelieveldt. Cardiac LV

segmentation using a 3D active shape model driven by fuzzy inference. In *Proc MICCAI*, volume 2878 of *LNCS*, pages 533–540. Springer, 2003.

[252] H. C. van Assen, M. G. Danilouchkine, A. F. Frangi, S. Ordás, J. J. M. Westenberg, J. H. C. Reiber, and B. P. F. Lelieveldt. SPASM: a 3D-ASM for segmentation of sparse and arbitrarily oriented cardiac MRI data. *Med Image Anal*, 10(2):286–303, Apr 2006.

[253] B. van Ginneken, M. de Bruijne, M. Loog, and M. A. Viergever. Interactive shape models. In M. Sonka and J. Fitzpatrick, editors, *Proc SPIE Medical Imaging*, volume 5032, pages 1206–1216, 2003.

[254] B. van Ginneken, A. F. Frangi, J. J. Staal, B. M. ter Haar Romeny, and M. A. Viergever. Active shape model segmentation with optimal features. *IEEE Trans Med Imaging*, 21(8):924–933, Aug 2002.

[255] B. van Ginneken, T. Heimann, and M. Styner. 3D segmentation in the clinic: A grand challenge. In T. Heimann, M. Styner, and B. van Ginneken, editors, *Proc MICCAI Workshop on 3D Segmentation in the Clinic*, pages 7–15, 2007.

[256] J. Vorsatz, C. Rössl, and H.-P. Seidel. Synamic remeshing and applications. *Journal of Computing and Information Science in Engineering*, 3(4):338–344, 2003.

[257] F. Vos, P. de Bruin, J. Aubel, G. Streekstra, M. Maas, L. van Vliet, and A. Vossepoel. A statistical shape model without using landmarks. In *Proc ICPR*, volume 3, pages 714–717, 23-26 Aug. 2004.

[258] Y. Wang, M.-C. Chiang, and P. M. Thompson. Automated surface matching using mutual information applied to Riemann surface structures. In *Proc MICCAI*, volume 3750 of *LNCS*, pages 666–674. Springer, 2005.

[259] Y. Wang, X. Gu, T. F. Chan, P. M. Thompson, and S.-T. Yau. Intrinsic brain surface conformal mapping using a variational method. In J. M. Fitzpatrick and M. Sonka, editors, *Proc SPIE Medical Imaging*, volume 5370, pages 241–252, 2004.

[260] Y. Wang, B. S. Peterson, and L. H. Staib. 3D brain surface matching based on geodesics and local geometry. *Comput Vis Image Underst*, 89:252–271, 2003.

[261] Y. Wang and L. H. Staib. Boundary finding with prior shape and smoothness models. *IEEE Trans Pattern Anal Mach Intell*, 22(7):738–743, July 2000.

[262] J. Weese, M. Kaus, C. Lorenz, S. Lobregt, R. Truyen, and V. Pekar. Shape constrained deformable models for 3D medical image segmentation. In *Proc IPMI*, volume 2082 of *LNCS*, pages 380–387. Springer, 2001.

[263] X. Wu and D. Z. Chen. Optimal net surface problems with applications. In *Proc. 29th Int'l Colloquium Automata, Languages, and Programming*, pages 1029–1042, 2002.

[264] P. Yu, P. Grant, Y. Qi, X. Han, F. Segonne, R. Pienaar, E. Busa, J. Pacheco, N. Makris, R. Buckner, P. Golland, and B. Fischl. Cortical surface shape analysis based on spherical wavelets. *IEEE Trans Med Imaging*, 26(4):582–597, April 2007.

[265] P. A. Yushkevich, H. Zhang, and J. C. Gee. Continuous medial representation for anatomical structures. *IEEE Trans Med Imaging*, 25(12):1547–1564, Dec. 2006.

[266] S. Zambal, J. Hladůvka, and K. Bühler. Improving segmentation of the left ventricle using a two-component statistical model. In *Proc MICCAI*, volume 4190 of *LNCS*, pages 151–158. Springer, 2006.

[267] Y. Zhan and D. Shen. Deformable segmentation of 3-D ultrasound prostate images using statistical texture matching method. *IEEE Trans Med Imaging*, 25:256–272, 2006.

[268] L. Zhang, H. Ai, S. Xin, C. Huang, S. Tsukiji, and S. Lao. Robust face alignment based on local texture classifiers. In *Proc ICIP*, volume 2, pages 354–357, 2005.

[269] Y. J. Zhang. A survey on evaluation methods for image segmentation. *Pattern Recognition*, 29(8):1335–1346, August 1996.

[270] M. Zhao, S. Z. Li, C. Chen, and J. Bu. Shape evaluation for weighted active shape models. In *Proc Asian Conference on Computer Vision*, volume 2, pages 1074–1079, Korea, January 2004.

*Bibliography*

[271] Z. Zhao, S. R. Aylward, and E. K. Teoh. A novel 3D partitioned active shape model for segmentation of brain MR images. In *Proc MICCAI*, volume 3749 of *LNCS*, pages 221–228. Springer, 2005.

[272] Z. Zhao and E. K. Teoh. A novel framework for automated 3D PDM construction using deformable models. In *Proc SPIE Medical Imaging*, volume 5747, pages 303–314, 2005.

[273] G. Zheng, K. Rajamani, X. Zhang, X. Dong, M. Styner, and L. Nolte. Kernel regularized bone surface reconstruction from partial data using statistical shape model. In *Proc Int Conf of the Engineering in Medicine and Biology Society*, pages 6579–6582, 01-04 Sept. 2005.

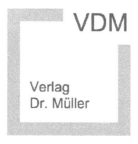

# Wissenschaftlicher Buchverlag bietet

kostenfreie

## Publikation

von

# wissenschaftlichen Arbeiten

Diplomarbeiten, Magisterarbeiten, Master und Bachelor Theses
sowie Dissertationen, Habilitationen und wissenschaftliche Monographien

Sie verfügen über eine wissenschaftliche Abschlußarbeit zu aktuellen oder zeitlosen
Fragestellungen, die hohen inhaltlichen und formalen Ansprüchen genügt,
und haben **Interesse an einer honorarvergüteten Publikation**?

Dann senden Sie bitte erste Informationen über Ihre Arbeit per Email
an info@vdm-verlag.de. Unser Außenlektorat meldet sich umgehend bei Ihnen.

VDM Verlag Dr. Müller Aktiengesellschaft & Co. KG
Dudweiler Landstraße 125a
D - 66123 Saarbrücken

www.vdm-verlag.de